Prevention of Falls and Hip Fractures in the Elderly

American Academy
of Orthopaedic Surgeons

Prevention of Falls and Hip Fractures in the Elderly

Edited by
David F. Apple, Jr., MD
Medical Director
Shepherd Spinal Center
Atlanta, Georgia

Wilson C. Hayes, PhD
Maurice E. Mueller Professor of Biomechanics
Harvard Medical School
Boston, Massachusetts

with 25 illustrations

Workshop
Westin Hotel O'Hare
Rosemont, Illinois
January 21-22, 1993

Supported by the
American Academy of Orthopaedic Surgeons

American Academy of Orthopaedic Surgeons
6300 North River Road
Rosemont, IL 60018

Prevention of Falls and Hip Fractures in the Elderly

Contributors and Workshop Participants

Itamar B. Abrass, MD†
Professor of Medicine
Head, Division of Gerontology and
  Geriatric Medicine
University of Washington
Seattle, Washington

Neal Alexander, MD*
Assistant Professor
Division of Geriatric Medicine
Department of Internal Medicine
University of Michigan
Ann Arbor, Michigan

Sharon A. Alleyne*
Director, Professional Relations and
  Education
National Osteoporosis Foundation
Washington, DC

David F. Apple, Jr., MD*†
Medical Director
Shepherd Spinal Center
Atlanta, Georgia

Timothy J. Bray, MD*
Associate, Reno Orthopaedic Clinic
Reno, Nevada

David M. Buchner, MD, MPH*†
Investigator, Northwest Health Services
  Research and Development Field
  Program
Seattle VA Medical Center
Seattle, Washington

Elizabeth Callan, MS†
Research Assistant
Department of Textiles and Clothing
Iowa State University
Ames, Iowa

James E. Carpenter, MD*†
Assistant Professor of Surgery
University of Michigan
Ann Arbor, Michigan

Mary Connolly*
Senior Program Specialist
American Association of Retired Persons
Washington, DC

Steven R. Cummings, MD†
Associate Professor of Medicine and
  Epidemiology
University of California
San Francisco, California

Thomas A. Einhorn, MD*†
Professor of Orthopaedics
Mount Sinai School of Medicine
New York, New York

Tobin N. Gerhart, MD†
Clinical Assistant Professor
Orthopaedic Surgery
Harvard Medical School
Boston, Massachusetts

Wilson C. Hayes, PhD*†
Maurice E. Mueller Professor of
  Biomechanics
Harvard Medical School
Boston, Massachusetts

Robert N. Hensinger, MD*
Professor, Section of Orthopaedics
University of Michigan
Ann Arbor, Michigan

Janet Hieshetter*
Director of Regional Services
National Osteoporosis Foundation
Washington, DC

Jeffrey C. Huston, PhD*†
Professor, Aerospace Engineering and
  Engineering Mechanics
Professor, Biomedical Engineering
Iowa State University
Ames, Iowa

C. Conrad Johnston, Jr., MD*†
Professor of Medicine
Chief, Division of Endocrinology and
  Metabolism
Indiana University School of Medicine
Indianapolis, Indiana

Patty Karlen, RN†
Project Director
Center for Health Studies
Group Health Cooperative
Seattle, Washington

Adam Karp, MD†
Clinical Instructor of Medicine
New York University School of Medicine
New York, New York

Thomas D. Koepsell, MD, MPH†
Professor and Chairman
Department of Epidemiology
Professor, Health Services
Adjunct Professor, Medicine
Co-Director, Robert Wood Johnson
   Clinical Scholars Program
University of Washington
Seattle, Washington

James C. Kudrna, MD, PhD*
Chief, Division of Orthopaedic Surgery
Evanston Hospital
Evanston, Illinois

Carolyn Kundel, PhD†
Associate Professor
Department of Textiles and Clothing
Iowa State University
Ames, Iowa

Lewis A. Lipsitz, MD*†
Usen Director of Medical Research
Hebrew Rehabilitation Center for Aged
Boston, Massachusetts

Joan A. McGowan, PhD*
Branch Chief
Bone Biology and Bone Diseases Branch
National Institute of Arthritis,
   Musculoskeletal and Skin Diseases
National Institutes of Health
Bethesda, Maryland

John N. Morris, PhD†
Director of Social and Health Policy
   Research
Co-Director, Research and Training
   Institute
Hebrew Rehabilitation Center for Aged
Boston, Massachusetts

Elizabeth R. Myers, PhD†
Assistant Professor
Department of Orthopaedic Surgery
Harvard Medical School
Boston, Massachusetts

Michael C. Nevitt, PhD*†
Associate Professor
Department of Epidemiology and
   Biostatistics
University of California at San Francisco
San Francisco, California

Jane Potts, CSW†
Social Worker
Hospital for Joint Diseases Orthopaedic
   Institute
New York, New York

Wayne A. Ray, PhD*
Professor of Preventive Medicine
Vanderbilt University School of Medicine
Nashville, Tennessee

William J. Robb, III, MD*
Clinical Assistant Professor
Department of Orthopaedic Surgery
Northwestern University Medical School
Chicago, Illinois

Mark Rosenberg, MD, MPP*†
Director, National Center for Injury
   Prevention and Control
Centers for Disease Control and
   Prevention
Atlanta, Georgia

Lisa Rubenstein, MHA*
Senior Program Specialist
American Association of Retired Persons
Washington, DC

Richard W. Sattin, MD, FACP*†
Chief, Scientific Review Section
National Center for Injury Prevention and
   Control
Centers for Disease Control and
   Prevention
Atlanta, Georgia

Michael S. Sellberg, MS†
Research Engineer
Department of Mechanical Engineering
Iowa State University
Ames, Iowa

Sherry Sherman, PhD*
Director, Osteoporosis Research
National Institute on Aging
National Institutes of Health
Bethesda, Maryland

Charles W. Slemenda, DrPH†
Associate Professor of Medicine
Indiana University School of Medicine
Indianapolis, Indiana

Peter G. Trafton, MD*†
Associate Professor
Department of Orthopaedics
Brown University
Providence, Rhode Island

Janet Weinstein, RN, NP†
Geriatric Falls Program
Hospital for Joint Diseases
New York, New York

Steven L. Wolf, PhD, FAPTA*†
Professor and Director of Research
Department of Rehabilitation Medicine
Professor of Geriatrics
Department of Medicine
Associate Professor
Department of Anatomy and Cell Biology
Emory University School of Medicine
Atlanta, Georgia

Harris S. Yett, MD†
Beth Israel Hospital
Boston, Massachusetts

Joseph D. Zuckerman, MD*†
Vice Chairman
Department of Orthopaedic Surgery
Hospital for Joint Diseases
New York, New York

*Workshop Participant
†Contributor to Volume

Preface

In 1989, the Committee on Rehabilitation, Prosthetics and Orthotics became interested in developing a workshop that would focus on balance training exemplified by "ball therapy" as a method to prevent falls. In 1991, the Board of Directors of the American Academy of Orthopaedic Surgeons funded a workshop to discuss prevention and rehabilitation disciplines on which the orthopaedist should focus more attention and energy. The focus of this workshop was the prevention of hip fractures secondary to falls in the elderly. The purpose of the workshop was to draw together the most significant researchers and clinicians concerned with the topic to discuss the status of knowledge, current treatment methods, and identification of future directions to bring the problem into proper perspective. Findings of the workshop are summarized in this monograph and provide the background for part of the Academy's three-pronged prevention initiative, Play It Safe, Live It Safe, and Work It Safe.

We thank the Academy for its support, the participants for their time and effort, and the orthopaedists who will read this monograph, take its concerns to heart, and transform those concerns into action.

We would like to thank Academy staff members involved in the organization of the workshop, Rebecca Maron, Director, Division of Health Policy, Scientific Affairs, and Communications; and Karen Schneider, Meetings Coordinator. Also, our appreciation is extended to Marilyn Fox, PhD, who directed the publications process, Lisa Claxton Moore, who managed the project and provided copy editing, and others on the production and editorial staff who worked to get this book published in a timely fashion.

David F. Apple, Jr., MD
Wilson C. Hayes, PhD

Table of Contents

Chapter 1

Injury Prevention: A National Perspective

Mark Rosenberg, MD, MPP

It is most exciting for me and for us at the Centers for Disease Control and Prevention (CDC) to be working in partnership with orthopaedists. George Bernard Shaw said that if you pay surgeons to cut off people's legs, that's what they'll do, but that's not what people want. What's striking to me about orthopaedists becoming involved in injury prevention is that they are looking at ways to avoid performing surgery for conditions that are avoidable. For many of us, especially those examining health care issues from a broad perspective, this attitude is very welcome.

At CDC, the nation's prevention agency, control of injury is focused on prevention. As the Clinton administration starts to look closely at health care costs, prevention is a logical consideration. They want to expand coverage to the many people who are not covered by the present system of health care. They want to both improve quality and cut down on the total cost. The only way to accomplish all three—cut costs, expand coverage, and improve quality—is to have effective prevention. Injury control has been relatively neglected as a research area but is one in which the benefits of prevention can be demonstrated.

In 1985, the National Academy of Sciences published a report called *Injury in America*. The committee who wrote the report was chaired by Bill Foege, a former director of CDC. According to this report, injury is the number one public health problem facing this country today and is so prevalent that one out of every four Americans is injured every year; however, it is a neglected field.

Injury is divided into three types by the CDC: motor vehicle, home and leisure, and intentional injuries (violence). Each injury type accounts for about one third (about 50,000 per year) of the total deaths attributed to injury. In 1993, the number of annual deaths from motor vehicle injuries fell below 40,000 for the first time. Home and leisure injuries include falls, which will be the focus of this presentation, and other unintentional injuries resulting from poisonings, drownings, fires, and burns.

Intentional injuries, or violence, can be separated into two types: interpersonal and self-directed. Interpersonal violence includes fatal injuries and nonfatal assaults. Included in this category are youth violence, child abuse, sexual assault, child sexual abuse, spousal violence, and elder abuse. Self-directed violence includes suicide and suicide attempts.

Although the focus of this publication is on falls among the elderly, I would like to mention children because they have been designated by the Clinton administration as an important health care focus. For people between ages 1 and 19, injuries account for more deaths than all diseases combined. One measure of the impact of any public health problem is years of potential life lost. Injury accounts for more years of potential life lost than any of the other leading causes of death for both children and adults and is the leading cause of death between ages 1 and 44.

Another measure of the impact of injury is the economic cost; injury in 1985 accounted for $158 billion in health care costs; in 1990, this figure is estimated at over $200 billion. This is a huge burden on the health care system. In 1985, there were a total of 142,000 fatal injuries; violence was the cause of about one third of these injuries. Injuries caused by firearms have been on the rise in this country since 1985 and are markedly increasing. The health care cost of injuries caused by firearms alone is estimated to be $14.4 billion in the United States. Those who work in a rehabilitation hospital know that more and more of the patients receiving rehabilitation have sustained injuries caused by firearms or other violence, especially in the inner cities.

The burden of intentional injury is particularly large among blacks. For young black males between the ages of 15 and 24, homicide is the leading cause of death (42%). What is less appreciated is that for young black women, homicide is also the leading cause of death. Our best information suggests that this problem is not so much associated with race, but is most closely associated with poverty, discrimination, and lack of opportunity. Homicide rates in the U.S. have increased markedly since 1986. An international comparison of homicide rates of the U.S. and 17 other industrialized countries shows that the U.S. rate for young white males exceeds the rates in all other countries; the rate for U.S. black males is extraordinarily high. These rates indicate the huge toll on our country's resources and shows the enormity of the effect of injury. Even though injury causes the loss of more years of potential life than cancer and heart disease combined, the resources and the attention given to injury are dwarfed by the resources given to cancer and cardiovascular diseases. Why is this? Perhaps because injuries have been viewed as accidents, as something that is inevitable, a part of our life. For example, because it is common for older people to fall and break the hip, these injuries have not attracted the attention of people focused on prevention. Another example is deaths on the highway. For some reason, people accept that deaths on the highway just happen as a cost of living in this modern world, but these deaths do not have to occur. If your young daughter is killed by a drunken driver, that's no accident. We can study the problem and find the causes. We can keep drunken drivers off the road. In Georgia, for example, there are many people who have been arrested three or more times for drunken driving. This death trap can be prevented.

The same principle applies to homicides. Young people have easier access to handguns, which increases the incidence of serious injury or death in this age group. Carjacking would not occur if the carjacker did not have a firearm or other weapon. This situation is preventable; we can make a difference by focusing on prevention. This is part of the conceptual change that needs to occur. In like manner, injuries resulting from falls in the elderly can be prevented; they do not have to be a leading cause of death for older people.

The issue of injury includes not only prevention but acute care and rehabilitation as well. The report, *Injury in America*, stated that no one brings together what can be learned from acute care and rehabilitation with what can be learned from prevention. There is no single focus in the country for this work. The CDC is attempting to bring together the experts in acute care and rehabilitation and fund research in these areas. People who care for patients in acute care and rehabilitation settings see how injuries occur, and this information can be very helpful for prevention. The CDC program divides injury control into prevention, acute care, and rehabilitation, the three phases of injury. In each of these areas, there are intramural programs and extramural research.

The CDC also builds programs in state and local health departments. Most state and local health departments have focused on traditional public health problems, such as salmonella risks in restaurants. They have not kept pace with the burden of illness or its prevention. The CDC is working with state health departments to enable them to look at injury control as a problem. Our center funds eight injury control research centers that bring together prevention of injuries, acute care, and rehabilitation in a number of different disciplines, such as engineering, rehabilitation, acute care, and physiology. The CDC also funds research project grants and individual RO1 grants in a number of different areas, and research program project grants that are individual grants on a common subject.

Some research findings that have resulted from this work have application for orthopaedics. Research on motorcycle helmets, for example, found that motorcycle crash death rates are 50% less in states with helmet laws. This kind of study, which is descriptive epidemiology of the problem, can be applied to fall injuries by looking at where fall injuries are less common. Are they equally common in different parts of the country? Are they less common in cold climates because people do not go out? Or are they more common in cold climates because people go out and slip on the ice? Are they more common where there is a population who exercises more? A number of facts can be considered—how rates vary in different places, how different laws affect rates, and how health care delivery systems impact on the changes in fall rates.

The use of bicycle helmets is an intervention that can be compared to a vaccine for head injuries. The main parallel is that wearing a bicycle helmet can reduce serious head injuries by 85%. What are the implications of that type of finding? First, people must wear the helmets. Similarly, it does no good to have a vaccine if children are not inoculated. An intervention doesn't prevent injury unless it is implemented, and right now the majority of children do not wear bicycle helmets. A few localities have passed mandatory bike helmet laws. For example, Howard County, Maryland, passed a law, and the usage rate went up from 4% to 47% in a very short period of time. New Jersey passed a mandatory bicycle helmet law for children. Passing mandatory-use laws is one way to get people to wear helmets.

How does this apply to preventing injuries from falls? It is not enough to develop interventions such as pads in underwear for older people that might prevent injuries from falls. People must use these devices. If it is known that better footwear can prevent falls, how can people be convinced to change systematically? How can those changes in behavior be encouraged? How can environmental modifications be made?

Some of our research at the CDC has suggested that playground surfaces are responsible for preventable injuries in children. Susan Baker, perhaps the founder of the modern era of injury control, illustrates this with the example of high metal sliding boards on playgrounds with concrete surfaces. Baker pointed out that the Occupational Safety and Health Administration would not allow anyone to work at that height on metal structures without a hard hat or a helmet. And yet we send little children up to that height. And, of course, they sometimes fall and are injured. Softer surfaces and lower heights for playground equipment can make a big difference in terms of injuries that occur here.

An obvious parallel to hip fractures is softer surfaces. But again the question comes up: if softer surfaces in homes or dwellings might be effective in preventing injury, how can they be put into place? Should there be a mandatory law? Should the Department of Housing and Urban Development establish these softer surfaces as requirements for building homes? How can these surfaces be tested to ensure their effectiveness?

It has been shown that medications used by the elderly may be associated with falls. How can this knowledge be applied? Which medications are involved and how significant is the risk of injury? Once these answers are found, how can physicians' prescribing and usage practices be changed to prevent those falls? Again, it is not enough to find out that medication is associated with falls.

Another example is handguns. The availability of handguns is a widespread problem; what interventions might be effective? Some very promising work has started to show that restrictive licensing of handguns can be effective in preventing injuries and deaths. For example, in Washington, DC, a law restricting handguns was very effective in reducing the death rate. This reduction is hard to see because the homicide rate in Washington is so high. But a sophisticated analysis by Colin Loftin at the University of Maryland that was published in the New England Journal of Medicine last year showed that the law, which forbade everyone except police and a few designated other groups to carry handguns, probably saved 47 lives a year over an 8-year period. That is a significant reduction. These laws work, and they can be quite effective.

The injury control community has worked to develop a national agenda for research and programs for injury control. Members of the orthopaedic community participated in this process, which included an agenda for preventing home and leisure injuries, which includes falls. At the CDC's national conference in Denver, agenda papers were presented and discussed, including the following topics: motor vehicle injuries, prevention of violence, home and leisure injuries, prevention of occupational injuries, trauma care, acute care systems, and rehabilitation. The CDC is now developing a national plan that will identify 22 (now completed) priorities for national injury control.

The results of a process such as this can be very important in helping to set priorities for research, not only what the CDC funds, but what the research agenda for the country should be. It can also have a significant impact on the availability of funding for research in this area. As previously mentioned, injury control is an emerging area and has not had as much attention from Congress or from the academic research institutions as other public health areas have. But that is starting to change.

A research and programmatic agenda concerning the prevention of falls created by orthopaedic surgeons would be helpful in identifying to Congress areas that need more funding.

There are a number of interventions that have proved effective in preventing injuries. At the CDC, we are writing a series of recommendations that it is hoped will help set national injury-control policy and will be supported by a number of other agencies. The first recommendation will be that bicycle helmets be worn at all times by bicycle riders. We hope that this recommendation will be used in much the same way that other CDC recommendations are used, for example, recommendations on immunizations, HIV infection, and National Institute for Occupational Safety and Health guidelines. It is hoped that the injury control guidelines will help develop and set policy. Other recommendations that will be developed will be on the use of motorcycle helmets, swimming pool fences, smoke detectors, sprinkler systems, sobriety checkpoints on the highways, and regulation of water heater temperature controls to prevent burns to children. Effective interventions need to be identified to prevent falls. Perhaps there will be recommendations for soft surfaces in private homes, nursing homes, or hospitals: for how patients should be moved from beds or kept in bed; or for hip padding for the elderly. Whatever the recommendations that might be forthcoming, there will be a mechanism for translating them into national policy.

The public health approach to dealing with health problems is a helpful framework for looking at the problem of preventing injuries from falls. This approach starts with defining the problem. What is known about it? How frequently does it occur? What are the risk factors and causes of this problem? With injuries resulting from falls, is osteoporosis a contributing factor? What is the contribution of different surfaces? What is the contribution of medication and drugs impairing an elderly person's ability to walk? What is the significance of how a person falls and grabs for support?

The next step is to develop and test interventions. What interventions look promising, and do they work? Evaluation research is very expensive. Often it is much cheaper to develop the intervention and then evaluate it. The next step is to get interventions into practice on a large scale, not just in the laboratory setting, perhaps in a community trial or even a statewide trial. And finally, the intervention must be implemented in the community or in the state to see how well it works. How is the intervention beneficial?

In conclusion, I think it is important that orthopaedists are examining the impact of falls and hip fractures in the elderly. As you know, it is a huge problem, but one for which prevention and development of intervention can make a difference.

Section One

Etiology: Intrinsic Factors

Chapter 2

Chronic Illness as a Risk Factor for Hip Fracture: Results of a Case-Control Study and Review of the Literature

David M. Buchner, MD, MPH
Thomas D. Koepsell, MD, MPH
Itamar B. Abrass, MD
Patty Karlen, RN

Introduction

A well-documented, dramatic increase in hip fracture incidence occurs in older adults.[1,2] The pathogenesis of hip fractures is recognized to be complex, involving a large number of risk factors. In discussing the role of disease (referred to as chronic conditions or chronic illness) as an etiologic factor, we begin with classification of risk factors for hip fracture. Next, we present data from a population-based case-control study, which found that about two thirds of patients with hip fracture have a chronic condition that reportedly increases fracture risk. Finally, we review the literature to show that our findings are typical of other studies. Our main theme is that hip fractures occur primarily in older adults with chronic illness, and in this sense, contribute to frail health in older adults.

Risk Factor Classification

Information about risk factors for hip fracture comes from a large number of epidemiologic studies—mainly case-control studies. The standard injury epidemiology model would classify the risk factors studied as either host, environment, or agent risk factors.[3] Diseases are clearly host risk factors. Because it is often hard to discern whether the disease, its treatment, or both are of etiologic importance, we prefer the term chronic conditions (or chronic illness) to refer to both diseases and treatment. Notably, we do not include age-related bone loss or osteoporosis as chronic conditions.

Almost all hip fractures in older adults occur as the result of a fall. Hence, risk factors for hip fracture can be further classified as to their mechanism of action, either to (1) increase fall risk, or (2) increase fracture risk when a fall occurs. Risk factors can act at either or both steps. Poor vision presumably increases hip fracture risk only by increasing fall risk. In contrast, bone weakness would logically only affect the risk of injury from a fall, and not fall risk. The same risk factor can operate at both steps in complementary or antagonistic ways. For example, muscle weakness is hypothesized to increase fall risk, and to increase fracture risk when a fall occurs. On the other hand, a thiazide diuretic may increase fall risk if it causes orthostatic hypotension, but decrease fracture risk because of an effect of thiazide diuretics on bone strength.[4] Almost all epidemiologic studies of hip fractures have selected controls irrespective of their fall history, and therefore summarize the combined effect of risk factors over the two steps.

Host risk factors can be further classified according to the conceptual framework of disability models. Consider the book, *Disability in America: Toward a National Agenda for Prevention*,[5] which proposed a model of disability involving pathophysiology (etiologic factors), physiologic impairments, functional limitations, and disability. The importance of this classification is its recognition of causal relationships among risk factors. For example, diabetes (an etiologic factor) can cause diabetic myopathy and muscle atrophy (a physiologic impairment), that in turn contributes to gait impairment (a functional limitation). Hence, the focus on chronic conditions is not meant to minimize the importance of physiologic impairments or functional limitations in the pathogenesis of hip fractures, but to improve understanding of what sort of health problems may be at the root of the hip fracture epidemic in older adults.

A Case-Control Study of the Role of Chronic Illness in Hip Fracture Risk

Methods

To clarify the importance of chronic conditions to hip fracture risk, we reviewed the literature to identify conditions thought to be related to hip fracture risk. Chronic conditions were grouped under the following categories: neurologic, musculoskeletal, systemic, and other major illnesses. Outline 1 provides the list of conditions.

We then performed a population-based, case-control study at a large HMO (Group Health Cooperative of Puget Sound) in Washington state. Hip fracture cases were prospectively identified over 21 months (n = 284). Controls were an age- and sex-stratified random

Outline 1 Categories of chronic illness

Neurologic conditions
  Global cognitive impairment (all causes)
  Other neurologic disease
    Stroke involving a leg
    Parkinson's disease
    Multiple sclerosis
    Polio involving a leg
    Cancer involving the brain
    Guillain-Barré syndrome involving a leg
Musculoskeletal conditions
  Amputation involving a leg
  Polymyalgia rheumatica
  Rheumatoid arthritis
  Heritable diseases of bone and muscle
  Paget's disease involving the hip
Systemic illnesses affecting bone metabolism
  Cushing's syndrome/chronic corticosteroid use
  Malabsorption syndromes
  Renal failure
  Cancer metastatic to bone
  Thyrotoxicosis
  Hyperparathyroidism
  Congenital hypogonadism
  Long-term heparin treatment
Other major illnesses
  Any illness causing inability to walk
  Any terminal illness

sample of 1,005 HMO enrollees, with 609 controls participating. Subjects were eligible for the study if they were at least 60 years old and spoke English.

Both cases and controls were screened for the illnesses. All cases were hospitalized at the time of the fracture, and we were able to screen almost 100% of cases using information in the hospital chart. However, we were concerned that mild dementia might not be noted in the hospital chart, or that temporary, postoperative delirium might be mistaken for dementia. Hence, four to six weeks after the fracture, we attempted to interview all patients using the Mini-Mental State Examination (MMSE).[6] However, only about 50% of cases agreed to be screened, so we may have underestimated the prevalence of dementia.

Because controls were not hospitalized, we used a different method of screening. First, HMO physicians identified some controls as having a chronic illness. Then, controls were screened by telephone for chronic illness. The third stage of screening was a clinic visit, where the MMSE was administered. In the screening, self report was deemed sufficient evidence of leg amputation, stroke, inability to walk, multiple sclerosis, Parkinson's disease, kidney failure, brain tumor, metastatic cancer, and polio. The medical chart was reviewed if a person claimed to have the following conditions: Guillain-Barré syndrome, steroid medication, rheumatoid arthritis, thyroid disease, parathyroid disease, adrenal disease, Paget's disease, polymyalgia rheumatica, malabsorption syndrome, chronic heparin treatment, or heritable disease of bone or muscle. In all, 609 of 1,005 controls were definitively screened, with the remaining 396 controls in the random sample declining study participation.

We were concerned that the controls who did not participate had more chronic conditions than the controls who participated. This situation would bias the study toward finding an association between chronic conditions and fracture risk. We used computerized medical records to compare the participating controls with the non-participants. Medication usage and hospitalization rates did not differ between groups. Primary care visits were more common in participants, possibly suggesting that participants were sicker. However, we suspect that the same factors leading the subjects to participate in the study also tend to increase outpatient utilization. The finding that participants are not sicker than nonparticipants, while perhaps nonintuitive, has been noted in other studies.[7,8] At any rate, the findings did not suggest that nonparticipation among potential controls would create a significant bias.

Using the known age and sex mix of the HMO population, it was possible to compute incidence rates of hip fracture. If one assumes that the prevalence of chronic conditions in the random sample control group is representative of the population, rates of hip fracture in adults can be calculated separately for adults with chronic illness, and for adults without. In this calculation, both the numerator and denominator of the rate are subject to sampling error, which must be taken into account in computing confidence intervals and performing statistical tests. Rates can then be used to calculate relative risks of hip fracture.

Results

The chronic conditions found in the 284 patients with hip fracture are shown in Table 1. Of these patients, 134 (47%) had a neurologic condition; of these 104 (37%) had cognitive impairment, and 27 (10%) had a stroke. About 6% of patients had rheumatoid arthritis or polymyalgia rheumatica. The two main systemic conditions affecting bone were chronic use of supraphysiologic corticosteroids and metastatic cancer. Finally, 10% of patients could not walk prior to the hip fracture. In total, 65% of patients had a chronic condition.

Table 2 shows that chronic illness was associated with increased hip fracture risk. Overall, the increase in risk in chronically ill HMO enrollees was more than fivefold, and was more dramatic in men (relative risk [RR] = 9.3) than in women (RR = 4.6).

Figure 1 shows the age- and sex-specific incidence rates of hip fracture at the HMO. The shapes of the curves closely resemble those of other populations, although rates are slightly lower than national rates.[1,2] Figure 2 shows incidence rates according to chronic illness status. Only a modest increase in hip fracture incidence with age oc-

Table 1 Prevalence of chronic illnesses in 284 consecutive hip fracture patients, as determined by concurrent medical record review*

Condition		N	Percent
Neurologic conditions		134	47%
Cognitive impairment		104	37%†
Other neurologic disease		40	14%
Stroke involving a leg	27		
Parkinson's disease	7		
Multiple sclerosis	2		
Polio involving a leg	2		
Cancer involving brain	1		
Guillain Barré syndrome	1		
Musculoskeletal conditions		17	6%
Polymyalgia rheumatica	7		
Rheumatoid arthritis	10		
Systemic conditions affecting bone		36	13%
Chronic use of corticosteroid drugs	20		
Malabsorption syndrome	1		
Chronic renal failure	1		
Metastatic cancer	19		
Other major illnesses		29	10%
Inability to walk	20		
Terminal illness	9		
Any of above		184	65%

*Categories are not mutually exclusive, so individual numbers do not necessarily sum to the totals shown.
†Note: 99 patients had medical record documentation of cognitive impairment; an additional 5 patients were classified as impaired based on a MMSE score below 25. Eighty-seven patients with a known chronic illness not including dementia, and 55 patients without a known chronic illness who refused to be interviewed, were not screened with the MMSE.

Table 2 Hip fracture risk associated with the presence of chronic illness

	Hip Fracture Incidence per 1,000 Patients Per Year		
	Chronic Illness (%)	No Chronic Illness (%)	Relative Risk (%) (95% Confidence Interval)
Women	19.0	2.3	4.6* (3.2 − 6.6)
Men	7.0	.46	9.3* (4.5 − 19.5)
All	13.3	1.4	5.3† (3.8 − 7.3)

*Relative risk adjusted for age.
†Relative risk adjusted for age and sex.

curred in women without chronic illness. Indeed, women age 85 and older without chronic illness had the same hip fracture rate as 65-year-old women with chronic illness. The most dramatic finding in Figure 2 was that hip fractures were unusual in men without chronic illness. In such men, aged 60 and older, the average hip fracture rate was quite low at 0.46/1,000/year (95% confidence interval $= 0.22 - 0.69$). The increased risk of fracture in older men with chronic illness was particularly dramatic.

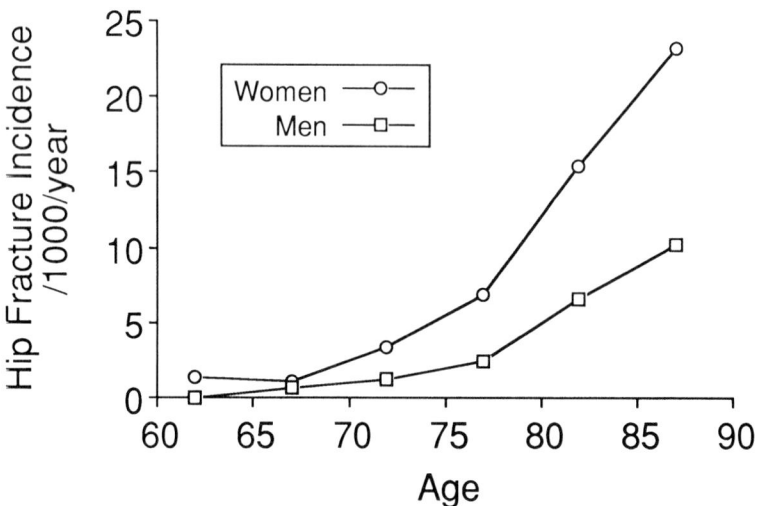

Fig. 1 *Annual age-specific incidence of hip fracture among HMO enrollees 60 years of age or older (N = 45,890) by gender (rates computed from 1987-1988 data).*

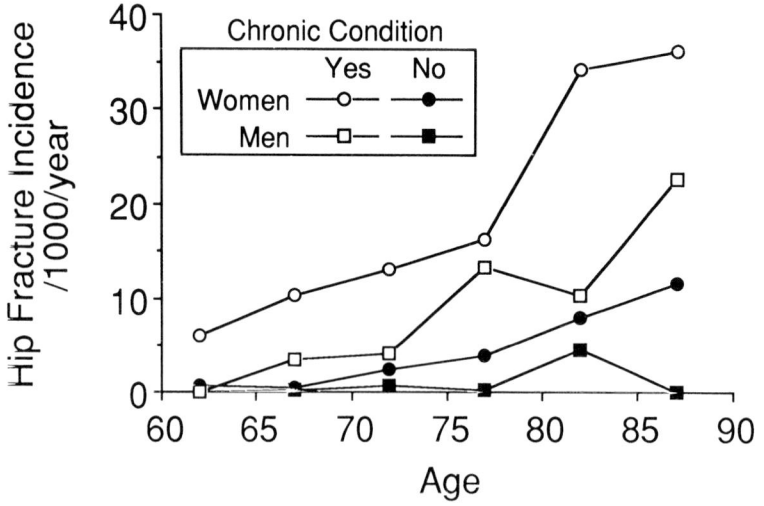

Fig. 2 *Annual age-specific incidence of hip fracture among HMO enrollees 60 years of age or older (N = 45,890) by gender and presence of chronic illness (rates computed from 1987-1988 data).*

Literature Review

The high prevalence of chronic conditions in the hip fracture cases noted in Table 1 is quite consistent with the published literature. As far back as 1955, Stewart[9] reported 58% of hip fracture patients had a serious illness. In 1962, Bauer[10] found a 41% prevalence of serious illness.

Dementia

Dementia is the most prevalent chronic condition in hip fracture patients. Prospective studies have estimated the prevalence of dementia as: 61%, >26%, 48%, 10%, >25%, 23%, and 40%,[11-17] with studies that carefully screen patients for dementia[11,17] estimating the higher rates. Presumably because mild dementia is not reliably detected, medical record studies have estimated a somewhat lower prevalence: 15%, 46%, 32%, and 20%.[18-21]

Further evidence of the importance of dementia as an etiologic factor in hip fracture comes from two cohort studies. One study found that patients with Alzheimer-type dementia have a 3.6-fold increase in hip fracture rates[22]; the other reported a 3.3-fold increase in risk.[23] Possibly, some of the association between dementia and fractures could be caused by the use of psychotropic drugs, which appear to increase fracture risk.[18,24] Because one study[22] involved a cohort that had been carefully screened for drug toxicity, and offending drugs were discontinued in another,[25] it is unlikely that this association can be accounted for by the high prevalence of psychotropic drug use in patients with dementia.

Other Conditions

Two recent studies[12,26] reported a prevalence of 6% and 4% of Parkinson's disease in hip fracture patients. Parkinson's disease was associated with a fourfold to sixfold increased risk of fracture, even after adjusting for a variety of confounders.[12,26]

The association of stroke with hip fracture risk has been known for some time, as fracture is more likely on the body side affected by the stroke. Reports of the prevalence of stroke in hip fracture cases are: 10%, 14%, 9%, and 17%.[16,27-29] In one study, stroke was associated with a 4.5-fold increase in fracture risk.[12] Two case-control studies have screened patients with hip fracture for rheumatoid arthritis, and found a prevalence of 14% and 24%.[27,28] A third study[30] of hip fractures and rheumatoid arthritis used a cohort design. The reported increased risk of hip fractures of approximately 1.5-fold in patients with rheumatoid arthritis was remarkably consistent across studies.

Finally, cancer and terminal illness are also probably prevalent in patients with hip fracture. For example, a recent study reported 15% of hip fracture patients were either terminally ill or had cancer.[12]

Summary

Chronic illness affects about two thirds of patients with hip fracture. These illnesses are not minor. Metastatic cancer, inability to walk, long-standing rheumatoid arthritis, and especially chronic degenerative neurologic disease such as dementia and stroke, are commonly present. These conditions are associated with increased risk of fracture, presumably by causing physiologic impairments such as bone weakness and functional limitations such as impaired gait, although the exact mechanisms have not been determined. Chronic illness may be a more important risk factor in men. In the reported case-control study, women with chronic illness had a 4.6-fold increase in fracture risk, whereas men with chronic illness had a 9.3-fold increase in fracture risk. Overall, the presence of a chronic condition increased risk about fivefold.

Hence, it is appropriate to regard hip fractures as part of the complex problem of frail health in older adults. While it is appropriate and important to focus on preventing hip fractures in healthy women, one should remember most hip fractures occur in adults who are chronically ill. Studies are needed of hip fracture prevention programs that target specific, high-risk subgroups. Interventions suitable for the general population may need substantial modification before they are applicable to some subgroups, such as patients with dementia. If future research confirms that healthy older men have a low fracture risk, the importance and priority of prevention efforts in this subgroup should be reconsidered.

References

1. Rodriguez JG, Sattin RW, Waxweiler RJ: Incidence of hip fractures, United States, 1970-83. *Am J Prev Med* 1989;5:175-181.
2. Jacobsen SJ, Goldberg J, Miles TP, et al: Hip fracture incidence among the old and very old: A population-based study of 745,435 cases. *Am J Public Health* 1990;80:871-873.
3. Waller JA: *Injury Control: A Guide to the Causes and Prevention of Trauma*. Lexington, MA, Lexington Books, 1985, chap 3, pp 11-38.
4. LaCroix AZ, Wienpahl J, White LR, et al: Thiazide diuretic agents and the incidence of hip fracture. *N Engl J Med* 1990;322:286-290.
5. Nagi SZ: Appendix A: Disability concepts revisited: Implications for prevention, in Pope AM, Tarlov AR (eds): *Disability in America: Toward a National Agenda for Prevention*. Washington, DC, National Academy Press, 1991, pp 309-327.
6. Folstein MF, Folstein SE, McHugh PR: "Mini-mental state": A practical method for grading the cognitive state of patients for the clinician. *J Psychiatr Res* 1975;12:189-198.
7. Wagner EH, Grothaus LC, Hecht JA, et al: Factors associated with participation in a senior health promotion program. *Gerontologist* 1991;31:598-602.
8. Durham ML, Beresford S, Diehr P, et al: Participation of higher users in a randomized trial of medicare reimbursement for preventive services. *Gerontologist* 1991;31:603-606.
9. Stewart IM: Fractures of the neck of the femur: Incidence and implications. *Br Med J* 1955;1:698-701.
10. Bauer GCH: Epidemiology of fracture in aged persons: A preliminary investigation in fracture etiology. *Clin Orthop* 1960;17:219-225.
11. Wood DJ, Cooper C, Stevens J, et al: Bone mass and dementia in hip fracture patients from areas with different aluminum concentrations in water supplies. *Age Ageing* 1988;17:415-419.
12. Grisso JA, Kelsey JL, Strom BL, et al: Risk factors for falls as a cause of hip fracture in women. *N Engl J Med* 1991;324:1326-1331.

13. Baker BR, Duckworth T, Wilkes E: Mental state and other prognostic factors in femoral fractures of the elderly. *J R Coll General Practitioners* 1978;28:557-559.

14. Magaziner J, Simonsick EM, Kashner TM, et al: Predictors of functional recovery one year following hospital discharge for hip fracture: A prospective study. *J Gerontol* 1990;45:M101-M107.

15. Cummings SR, Phillips SL, Wheat ME, et al: Recovery of function after hip fracture: The role of social supports. *J Am Geriatr Soc* 1988;36:801-806.

16. Campion EW, Jette AM, Cleary PD, et al: Hip fracture: A prospective study of hospital course, complications, and costs. *J Gen Intern Med* 1987;2:78-82.

17. Billig N, Ahmed SW, Kenmore P, et al: Assessment of depression and cognitive impairment after hip fracture. *J Am Geriatr Soc* 1986;34:499-503.

18. Ray WA, Griffin MR, Schaffner W, et al: Psychotropic drug use and the risk of hip fracture. *N Engl J Med* 1987;316:363-369.

19. Schorr RI, Griffin MR, Daugherty JR, et al: Opioid analgesics and the risk of hip fracture in the elderly: Codeine and propoxyphene. *J Gerontol* 1992;47:M111-M115.

20. Matheny L II, Scott TF, Craythorne CM, et al: Hospital mortality in 342 hip fractures. *West Virginia Med J* 1980;76:188-190.

21. Clayer MT, Bauze RJ: Morbidity and mortality following fractures of the femoral neck and trochanteric region: Analysis of risk factors. *J Trauma* 1989;29:1673-1678.

22. Buchner DM, Larson EB: Falls and fractures in patients with Alzheimer-type dementia. *JAMA* 1987;257:1492-1495.

23. Morris JC, Rubin EH, Morris EJ, et al: Senile dementia of the Alzheimer's type: An important risk factor for serious falls. *J Gerontol* 1987;42:412-417.

24. Ray WA, Griffin MR, Downey W: Benzodiazepines of long and short elimination half-life and the risk of hip fracture. *JAMA* 1989;262:3303-3307.

25. Larson EB, Kukull WA, Buchner D, et al: Adverse drug reactions associated with global cognitive impairment in elderly persons. *Ann Intern Med* 1987;107:169-173.

26. Hammer AJ: Intertrochanteric and femoral neck fractures in patients with parkinsonism. *S African Med J* 1991;79:200-202.

27. Stevens A, Mulrow C: Drugs affecting postural stability and other risk factors in the hip fracture epidemic: Case-control study. *Community Med* 1989;11:27-34.

28. Gallagher JC, Melton LJ, Riggs BL: Examination of prevalence rates of possible risk factors in a population with a fracture of the proximal femur. *Clin Orthop Rel Research* 1980;153:158-165.

29. Clark AN: Factors in fracture of the female femur: A clinical study of the environmental, physical, medical and preventive aspects of this injury. *Geront Clin* 1968;10:257-270.

30. Hooyman JR, Melton LJ III, Nelson AM, et al: Fractures after rheumatoid arthritis: A population-based study. *Arthritis Rheum* 1984;27:1353-1361.

Chapter 3

The Roles of Osteoporosis and Falls in Hip Fractures in the Elderly

Thomas A. Einhorn, MD

Fracture of the hip is one of the most common and medically devastating conditions afflicting older persons, threatening survival as well as independence. This year, 280,000 Americans will suffer hip fractures and by current estimates, this number will climb to 340,000 in the year 2000, and 650,000 in the year 2050.[1] Eighty-seven percent of hip fracture patients are 65 years of age or older and 75% are women.[1] By age 90, it is expected that 33% of women and 15% of men will have had at least one hip fracture.[2] Of these, from 5% to 25% of patients will have died within three months following surgery to repair the fractured hip.[1] Nationwide, the annual cost of treating hip fractures is nearly $10 billion.[3]

Although multiple factors contribute to the occurrence of hip fracture, osteoporosis and falls are clearly the most significant. While the relative contribution of each of these factors to hip fracture incidence remains controversial, most investigators agree that a combination of factors is generally required in order for a hip fracture to occur. The relevant issues for the genesis of hip fractures in the elderly are (1) whether or not a fall occurs; (2) the mechanism of the fall; and (3) how well bones and soft tissues can absorb the energy of an impact once a fall is initiated.

Causes and Conditions in Falls

It has been estimated that approximately 90% of hip fractures occur as a result of a fall and approximately 10% occur spontaneously.[2] Although only 19% of falls in the elderly lead to hip fracture, falls are the leading cause of hip fracture.[2] Because most hip fractures occur at home, resulting from hazards such as throw rugs, poorly lit stairways, slippery bathtubs, and electrical cords, measures to modify the home environment could have a major positive effect in reducing the overall incidence of falls. In general, falls in the elderly are caused by age-related impairments in neuromuscular, cardiac, and cerebral function.[4] For example, cardiac insufficiency can result in temporary dizziness upon arising from a prone position. Irregular heart rhythms can also lead to brief episodes of unconsciousness. Other conditions that contribute to an increased incidence of falls include poor eyesight, foot problems, and severe arthritic conditions that impair gait and balance.[5] Because these factors are significantly heterogeneous, the prevention of falls in the elderly remains a complex problem.

Between the time that an individual begins to fall and the time they strike the ground, several factors may come into play that could influence whether or not a hip fracture results (Fig. 1). These factors include the orientation of the faller, the faller's protective response, local shock absorbers, protective garments, local environment, and the material and structural properties of the bones that form the hip joint.[6]

The orientation of the faller can largely affect the outcome of the fall in terms of the type of injury sustained. For example, a fall backward, landing on the buttock, may be a reasonably safe mechanism for falling and often leads to only minimal trauma.[7] A fall forward, landing on the outstretched hand, generally can protect the hip joint from fracture but may lead to a fracture of the distal radius (Colles' fracture).[7] A fall to the side is reportedly associated with the highest incidence of hip fractures, and studies have demonstrated that even physically fit, conditioned athletes have difficulty breaking their fall while in this position.[8]

One of the biggest problems with falls in the elderly is the inability of the faller to mount a protective response. In younger individuals, the protective response frequently leads to an avoidance of injury. However, studies have shown that between the ages of 65 and 85 there is a 20% to 30% decrease in reaction time.[6] In addition, substances such as cigarette smoke and alcohol impair the protective response. Because it is well known that elderly individuals, in compromised states of health, may require certain pharmacologic agents, an understanding of the potential side effects of these agents is required. For example, long-acting hypnotic drugs such as flurazepam, diazepam, and chlordiazepoxide, which are often prescribed to elderly patients with insomnia, depression, or anxiety, are associated with a diminished protective response[9] and can lead to dizziness and impaired balance. In addition, narcotic analgesics, cyclic antidepressants, a variety of anticonvulsants, and antihypertensives may be associated with an increased incidence of falls.[10-12]

Local shock absorbers may play an important role in preventing the occurrence of hip fracture. Studies have shown that thinner women, with less adipose tissue between the greater trochanter and skin, have double the risk of hip fracture when compared with average-sized or obese women.[2,4] Moreover, muscle strength in the hip

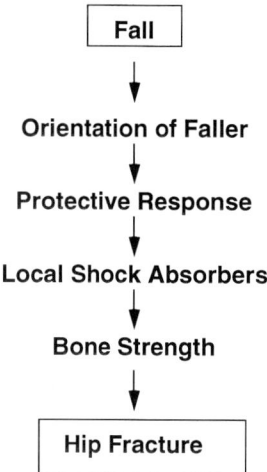

Fig. 1 *Flow diagram demonstrating the factors that could influence a hip fracture outcome as the result of a fall. (Adapted with permission from Cummings SR, Nevitt MC: A hypothesis: The causes of hip fractures. J Gerontol 1989;44:M107-M111.)*

abductors has been shown to undergo a 20% decline between the ages of 60 and 85, and the ability of these muscles to absorb energy has been shown to be significant.[2,6] Recent studies show that garments that pad the hip can help prevent hip fractures that result from falls.[13]

Role of Osteoporosis in the Etiology of Hip Fractures: Review of the Evidence

The role of osteoporosis in the etiology of hip fractures remains unclear. There seems to be little doubt that a reduction in bone's mechanical properties places the hip at increased risk for fracture. However, the extent to which osteoporosis may be involved in causing hip fractures in the elderly remains to be demonstrated. While osteoporosis is presently defined as a "decrease in the amount of bone leading to an increase in fracture risk,"[3] the events that lead to the actual hip fracture have not yet been determined.

Several investigators have examined whether osteoporotic patients are at increased risk for hip fracture. In his review of 15 case control studies, Cummings[14] concluded that patients with hip fractures do not appear to have significantly more osteoporotic bone than persons of similar age without fractures, and that factors other than bone mass (such as tendency to fall) may be more important predictors of which patients will fracture their hips.[14] In a more recent report (in which Cummings was a co-investigator), one of many to flow from a large prospective cohort study, 9,704 non-African American women 65 years of age or older were studied. These patients were recruited from a population-based listing of four clinical centers: the Kaiser-Permanente Center for Health Research in Portland, Oregon, the University of Minnesota in Minneapolis, the University of Maryland in Baltimore, and the Monongahela Valley, Pennsylvania area as part of the Study of Osteoporotic Fractures Multicenter Research Group project. By measuring bone mass at the distal and proximal radius, as well as the calcaneus, using single photon absorptiometry, these investigators concluded that most types of skeletal fractures do have an increased incidence in elderly women with low bone mass.[15] Moreover, it was shown that bone mineral density measurements at any one of three commonly used sites in the appendicular skeleton (distal radius, proximal radius, or calcaneus) have essentially the same predictive value in determining the risk of hip fracture within the next 0.8 to 2.8 years. A decrease in bone mineral density at any one of these sites of one standard deviation below the mean at all determinations, adjusted for age, predicts a 50% increase for hip fracture.[16]

One potential problem in determining how osteoporosis affects fracture incidence may be related to the definition of what constitutes osteoporosis on the basis of bone density. This may be partially related to the fact that the presence of osteoporosis requires not only "low bone mass" but also "increased fracture risk." Because the geometry and architecture of bone may largely dictate which bones with low bone mass are going to fracture, the ability of bone density measurements to make these predictions may be in question.[17] Nevertheless, most bone density measurements taken at the level of the hip are reported by comparing the patient's bone density to that of other patients of the same age. Bone density that is less than one standard deviation from the norm for the patient's age suggests that the risk of hip fracture is low. However, it has been suggested that a fracture threshold for the hip exists and any bone density below this level increases the risk of fracture. Figure 2 shows a bone density study using dual energy x-ray absorptiometry at the hip in a patient whose bone mineral density is squarely within the normal range for age. However, the fracture threshold is above this patient's bone density, thus placing the hip within the range of fracture risk. Moreover, because this patient's bone mineral density is normal for age but 2.5 standard deviations below that of younger, normal individuals, her risk for developing a hip fracture is 20 times that of young normal women.

Greenspan and associates[18] have recently examined femoral bone density as a potential predictor of hip fractures in fallers. Bone mineral density was evaluated by dual energy x-ray absorptiometry and bone mass index in 182 fallers who were older than 65 years. Femoral bone density was also determined in the contralateral hip of

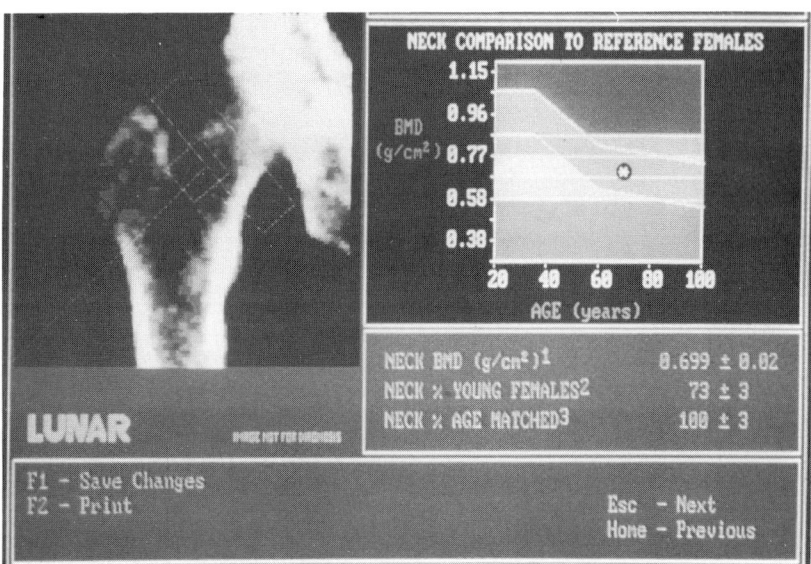

Fig. 2 *Dual energy x-ray absorptiometry report of the bone density in a 70-year-old woman. The asterisk on the graph shows the patient's bone density, which is approximately 0.70 g/cm². This density is in the center of the range of normal values for the patient's age; however, it is below the "fracture threshold," which is estimated to be at 0.77 g/cm². Moreover, because the bone density is 2.5 standard deviations below that of young normal individuals, her risk of developing a hip fracture is 20 times that of a young normal woman. (Reproduced with permission from the Lunar Corporation, Madison, WI.)*

patients less than one week after fracture. The investigators showed that the most important determinant of hip fracture for both men and women was bone mineral density at the femoral neck. They concluded that, in fallers whose bone mineral density is already below the fracture threshold, measurements of femoral neck bone mineral density can distinguish fallers who fracture a hip from those who do not.[18]

Bone Loss at the Hip and Relationship to the Type of Hip Fracture Sustained

Although most reports addressing the relationship between hip fracture and osteoporosis have grouped all fractures under one general heading, at least three different types of hip fractures exist and the anatomic, biomechanical, and biologic considerations underlying their occurrence and healing capabilities are distinct. Figure 3 shows the three basic types of proximal femur (hip) fractures. The intracapsular fracture (otherwise known as femoral neck or transcervical fracture) occurs through an area whose cross-section is composed of

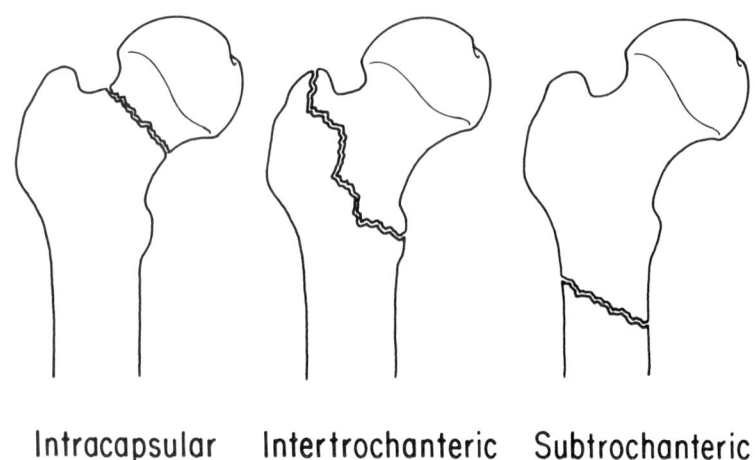

Intracapsular   Intertrochanteric   Subtrochanteric

Fig. 3 *The three types of proximal femur fractures.*

at least 75% cortical bone. On the other hand, the intertrochanteric fracture occurs through an area composed of approximately 50% trabecular bone. Moreover, because the stresses in the femur change along a proximal to distal gradient,[19] the biomechanical load at each of these sites will also differ. Because the majority of hip fractures occurring in the elderly are either intracapsular or intertrochanteric, the remainder of this discussion will focus on these two types.

It is generally believed that areas of the skeleton that undergo fracture associated with low bone mass are those that are largely composed of trabecular bone. In these areas, horizontal trabeculae are lost as a consequence of aging, and this leads to an alteration in the mechanical competence of the skeleton.[20] The vertebrae, distal radius, and intertrochanteric regions of the femur are at risk for sustaining fractures as a result of postmenopausal or age-associated trabecular bone loss.[15] Because trabecular bone has approximately eight times the remodeling rate of cortical bone, dysfunctional metabolic states such as those that occur as a result of hyperthyroidism, glucocorticoid use, and, in certain women, menopause, may lead to osteoporosis at these sites.[21] On the other hand, it is well known that as a result of endosteal resorption and periosteal apposition, diaphyseal sections of the long bones increase in diameter with age; the cortical compartments of most long bones become thinner, but the overall diameters increase.[22,23] Because bending strength, torsional strength, and areal and polar moments of inertia are related to the cross-sectional diameters of the long bones, all of these biomechanical properties are increased as a result of cross-sectional expansion. The skeleton has developed a protective mechanism as a result of geometric changes, and this may compensate for the loss of tissue-level protection that results from cortical thinning. Based on this knowledge, and considering the fact that the femoral neck is composed of 75% cortical bone, this anatomic site would not be expected to be at risk for hip fractures. Nevertheless, intracapsular fractures occur with nearly the same incidence as intertrochanteric fractures.[24,25]

To understand the etiology of intracapsular versus intertrochanteric fractures, Uitewaal and associates[24] histomorphometrically analyzed transilial bone biopsies from 39 hip fracture patients, 21 of whom had femoral neck fractures and 18 of whom had intertrochanteric fractures. They concluded that the intertrochanteric fractures were associated with osteoporosis but the intracapsular fractures represented a more heterogeneous group. Vega and associates[25] found similar results using photon densitometry.

The explanation for these findings may be that the femoral neck is not protected by the same cortical expansion mechanism as the remainder of the skeleton. Because the hip capsule inserts at the most distal part of the femoral neck (Fig. 4), and because the bone within the hip joint is not invested with an osteoprogenitor cell-rich cambium layer in its periosteum,[26,27] cortical bone in the femoral neck may undergo endosteal resorption without the benefit of compensatory periosteal apposition. This could lead to cortical thinning without an associated change in cross-sectional diameter.[23] As a result, biomechanical protection would not be afforded to the femoral neck as it would for the diaphyseal parts of long bones.

As discussed, areas of the skeleton largely composed of trabecular bone, such as the trochanteric region of the femur, are at risk for reduced mechanical competence when bone loss occurs. In general, this bone loss is attributed to the aging process or the postmenopausal state; however, certain endocrine conditions can lead to an acceleration of the uncoupling of bone resorption to formation in favor of bone loss. A recent report by Bauer and associates[28] showed that hyperthyroidism increases the risk of hip fracture. This investigation, which was part of the Study of Osteoporotic Fractures Multicenter Research Group project, assessed the history of hyperthyroidism and use of thyroid hormone in this large cohort of patients. After adjusting for age, weight, and change in weight since age 35, current use of thyroid supplement was associated with an increased risk of hip fracture. These investigators concluded that hyperthyroidism, either endogenous or exogenous, substantially increases the risk of hip fracture and the mechanism may be independent of bone mass.[28] Why this occurs independent of bone mass is not clear, but it may be related to a mechanical state induced by the high remodeling conditions present in bone exposed to significant levels of thyroid hormone. If the normal homeostatic mechanisms that maintain bone quality can be correlated with those that ensure the integrity of a mechanical structure, a useful analogy can be developed. Consider two brick walls, one that undergoes controlled repair and remodeling while the other is continuously being patched in order to keep

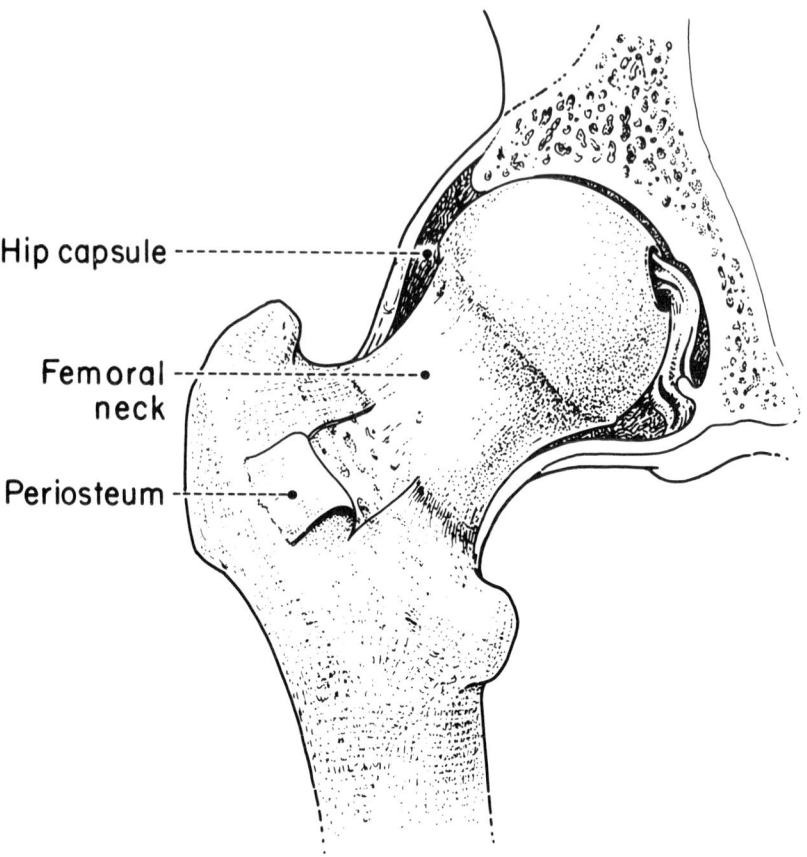

Fig. 4 *Anatomic drawing of the proximal femur and hip joint. Note that the hip capsule inserts at the base of the femoral neck and defines the distal boundary of the hip joint. The proximal edge of the periosteal covering of the femur ends at the point where the hip capsule inserts, leaving the bone of the femoral neck (intracapsular) devoid of periosteum.*

pace with its chronic degeneration (Fig. 5). Both structures may have the same mass but the one that is constantly being excavated and repaired is weaker mechanically. In the case of bone, when osteoclastic resorption is followed by osteoblastic formation in a rapid, chaotic state, poor bone quality will result despite no net change in bone mass.

Stress Fractures of the Hip

Fractures occur as a result of static load or repetitive stress. Although the majority of fractures are the result of static load (a person sustains an impact to the hip, causing it to break), stress fractures may account for as many as 10% of the fractures in the proximal femur.

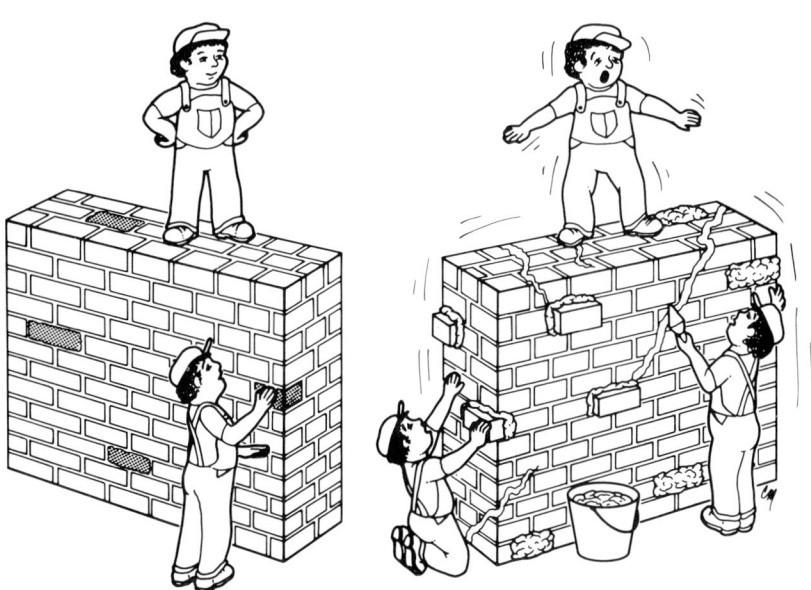

Fig. 5 *Cartoon demonstrating that two brick walls of the same mass and dimensions will have different mechanical properties if one is constantly being excavated and patched whereas the other undergoes controlled remodeling. This situation may be analogous to bone that is in a state of high turnover versus bone that experiences normal homeostatic remodeling. (Reproduced with permission from Einhorn TA: Bone strength: The bottom line.* Calcif Tissue Int *1992;51:333-339.)*

Stress fractures can be broadly divided into three types: pathologic, fatigue, and insufficiency fractures.[29] Pathologic fractures occur in diseased bone and the term is generally reserved for fractures through primary bone tumor or bony tumor metastases. Because these conditions are not directly relevant to the current discussion, pathologic fractures will not be reviewed here. In fatigue fractures, normal bone is subjected to greater than normal stress. These fractures are usually seen in unseasoned military recruits and athletes in training who undergo activity to which they are not accustomed. Insufficiency fractures are the ones most commonly seen in elderly patients with low bone mass. Here, failure occurs either as a result of decreased elastic resistance of bone or an accumulation of microfractures.[30] It is postulated that, in certain patients, the intrinsic ability of the femoral neck to withstand loading diminishes to a level below that of the daily stress to which it is exposed. Trabecular microfractures then begin and fracture propagation ensues.[31] Figure 6, *left* shows an intact proximal femur with a radiodense line across the femoral neck. A technetium 99mDP bone scan (Fig. 6, *right*) shows increased isotopic uptake in this area. Microscopically, the increased density is most likely caused by the accumulation of numerous tra-

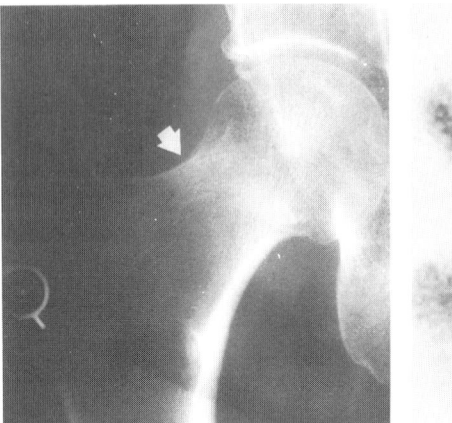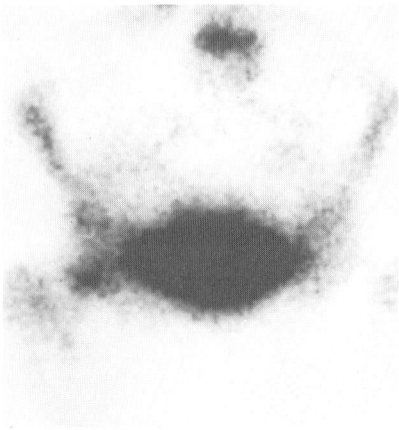

Fig. 6 *Left,* Radiograph of the proximal femur in a patient with gradually progressing pain in the groin. The arrow demonstrates a subtle radiodense line across the femoral neck. ***Right,*** *Technetium 99mDP bone scan in this patient shows increased isotopic uptake in the area of the femoral head and neck.*

becular microfractures healed by microcalluses (Fig. 7). Based on these observations, it is apparent that any delay or interference in the healing of these microfractures could lead to a mechanically compromised femoral neck. Examples of conditions that could alter microfracture healing include pituitary dysfunction,[32] sodium fluoride use,[33,34] and possibly, prolonged estrogen deficiency.[35] Recently, Lucas and Einhorn[36] observed that the combination of increased repetitive stress in a patient who had been taking glucocorticoids and immunosuppressive drugs led to the development of a femoral neck stress fracture. They hypothesized that the ability of the skeleton to adapt to an acute alteration in mechanical loading patterns was impaired by the presence of pharmacologic agents that altered bone metabolism.[36]

Hip Fracture Prevention Strategies

Prevention of disease is a much more effective treatment strategy than pursuit of a medical cure. With hip fractures, several causes have been identified. Efforts to modify drug and alcohol use and cigarette smoking could potentially lead to a reduction in the number of hip fractures. Likewise, strategies to prevent falls, such as improving protective responses and gait, increasing muscle strength and tone, and enrolling elderly patients in carefully designed rehabilitation programs, could be effective. Efforts to "accident-proof" the home environment would also seem to be a reasonable approach to this problem.

There appears to be good evidence that certain nutritional and pharmacologic treatments can prevent hip fracture rates. Kiel and as-

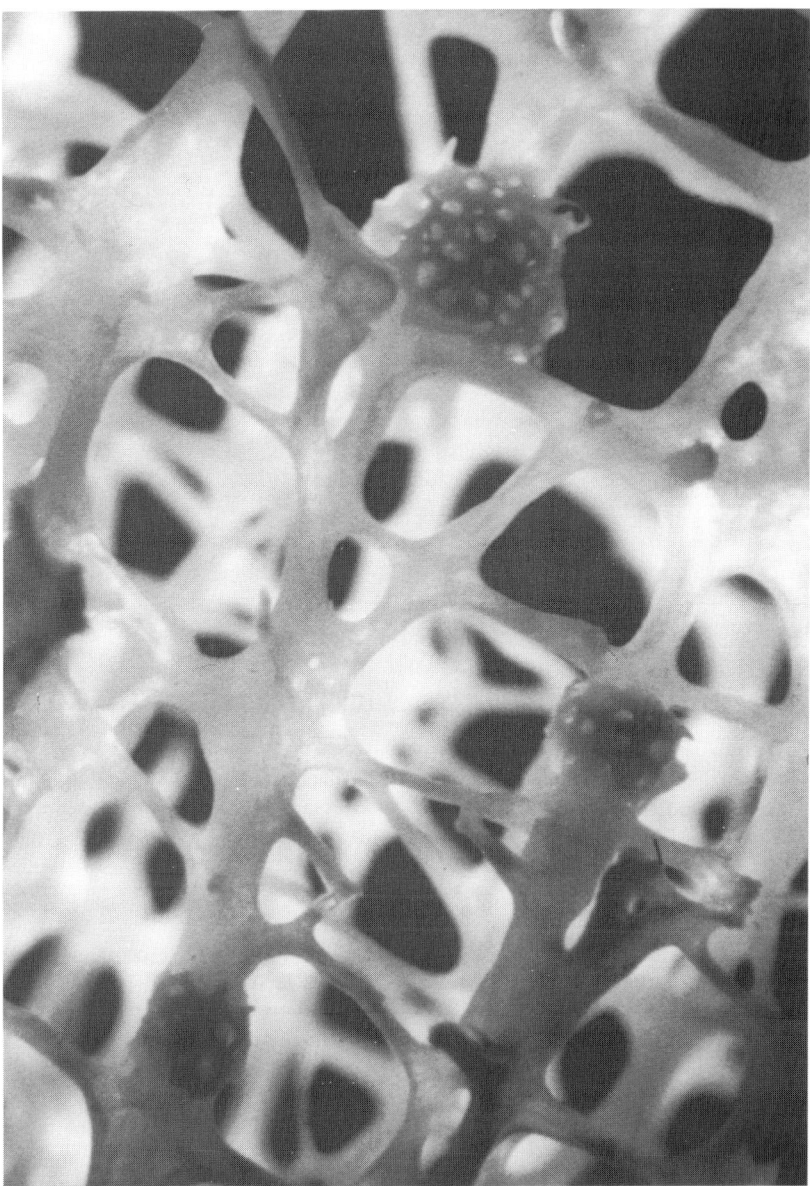

Fig. 7 *Close-up photograph of trabecular bone showing the accumulation of numerous microfractures that have healed with the formation of microcalluses. (Reproduced with permission from Klein MJ: Microtrabecular fractures: Lumbar vertebra. Lab Med 1991;22:654.)*

sociates[37] studied hip fractures in women in the Framingham Heart Study and examined these individuals for estrogen use as well as smoking habit. They showed that five years of estrogen use reduced both hip fracture and cardiac mortality rates by more than 50% in nonsmokers or former smokers.[37] Vitamin D and calcium have also been shown to protect against hip fractures. Chapuy and associates[38] studied the effects of supplementation with vitamin D3 and calcium on the frequency of hip fractures and other nonvertebral fractures in 3,270 healthy women with an average age of 84 ± 6 years. Among the women who completed the 18-month study, the number of hip fractures was 43% lower and the total number of nonvertebral fractures was 32% lower in the women who were treated with vitamin D3 and calcium when compared to those who were not. These investigators concluded that supplementation with vitamin D and calcium reduces the risk of hip fractures and other nonvertebral fractures among elderly women.[38]

Other measures to prevent hip fracture incidence are currently under investigation. As discussed, the use of hip pads and related protective devices may prove to be effective in the long run. Because of the vast impact of the potential hip fracture epidemic on our increasing elderly population, any measure that can significantly reduce hip fracture incidence will most certainly lead to the savings of billions of dollars, and hopefully, thousands of lives.

References

1. Brody JA: Prospects for an ageing population. *Nature* 1985;315:463-466.
2. Cummings SR, Kelsey JL, Nevitt MC, et al: Epidemiology of osteoporosis and osteoporotic fractures. *Epidemiol Rev* 1985;7:178-208.
3. Riggs BL, Melton LJ III: The prevention and treatment of osteoporosis. *N Engl J Med* 1992;327:620-627.
4. Tinetti ME, Speechley M, Ginter SF: Risk factors for falls among elderly persons living in the community. *N Engl J Med* 1988;319:1701-1707.
5. Grisso JA, Kelsey JL, Strom BL, et al: Risk factors for falls as a cause of hip fracture in women: The Northeast Hip Fracture Study Group. *N Engl J Med* 1991;324:1326-1331.
6. Cummings SR, Nevitt MC: A hypothesis: The causes of hip fractures. *J Gerontol* 1989;44:M107-M111.
7. Nevitt MC: Characteristics of falls and fallers and the risk of hip and wrist fracture, in Apple DF Jr, Hayes WC (eds): *Prevention of Falls and Hip Fractures in the Elderly*. Rosemont, IL, American Academy of Orthopaedic Surgeons, 1994, chap 6.
8. Van den Kroonenberg A, Munih P, Weigent-Hayes M, et al: Hip impact velocities and body configurations for experimental falls from standing height. *Trans Orthop Res Soc* 1993;18:24.
9. Gerhart TN: Managing and preventing hip fractures in the elderly. *J Musculoskeletal Med* 1987;4:60-68.
10. Ray WA, Griffin MR, Schaffner W, et al: Psychotropic drug use and the risk of hip fracture. *N Engl J Med* 1987;316:363-369.
11. Ray WA, Griffin MR, Downey W, et al: Long-term use of thiazide diuretics and risk of hip fracture. *Lancet* 1989;1:687-690.
12. LaCroix AZ, Wienpahl J, White LR, et al: Thiazide diuretic agents and the incidence of hip fracture. *N Engl J Med* 1990;322:286-290.

13. Huston JC, Sellberg MS, Kundel C, et al: A passive protective device to prevent hip fracture from falls in the elderly, in Apple DF Jr, Hayes WC (eds): *Prevention of Falls and Hip Fractures in the Elderly*. Rosemont, IL, American Academy of Orthopaedic Surgeons, 1994, chap 13.

14. Cummings SR: Are patients with hip fractures more osteoporotic? Review of the evidence *Am J Med* 1985;78:487-494.

15. Seeley DG, Browner WS, Nevitt MC, et al: Which fractures are associated with low appendicular bone mass in elderly women? The Study of Osteoporotic Fractures Research Group. *Ann Intern Med* 1991;115:837-842.

16. Cummings SR, Black DM, Nevitt MC, et al: Appendicular bone density and age predict hip fracture in women: The Study of Osteoporotic Fractures Research Group. *JAMA* 1990;263:665-668.

17. Einhorn TA: Bone strength: The bottom line. *Calcif Tissue Int* 1992;51:333-339.

18. Greenspan SL, Maitland LA, Myers ER, et al: Femoral bone density: A predictor of hip fracture in fallers. *J Bone Miner Res* 1992;7:S121.

19. Fielding JW, Cochran GV, Zickel RE: Biomechanical characteristics and surgical management of subtrochanteric fractures. *Orthop Clin North Am* 1974;5:629-650.

20. Mosekilde L, Viidik A, Mosekilde L: Correlation between the compressive strength of iliac and vertebral trabecular bone in normal individuals. *Bone* 1985;6:291-295.

21. Parfitt AM, Mathews CH, Villanueva AR, et al: Relationships between surface, volume, and thickness of iliac trabecular bone in aging and in osteoporosis: Implications for the microanatomic and cellular mechanisms of bone loss. *J Clin Invest* 1983;72:1396-1409.

22. Smith RW Jr, Walker RR: Femoral expansion in aging women: Implications for osteoporosis and fractures. *Henry Ford Hosp Med J* 1980;28:168-170.

23. Ruff CB, Hayes WC: Subperiosteal expansion and cortical remodeling of the human femur and tibia with aging. *Science* 1982;217:945-948.

24. Uitewaal PJ, Lips P, Netelenbos JC: An analysis of bone structure in patients with hip fracture. *Bone Miner* 1987;3:63-73.

25. Vega E, Mautalen C, Gomez H, et al: Bone mineral density in patients with cervical and trochanteric fractures of the proximal femur. *Osteoporosis Int* 1991;1:81-86.

26. Pankovich AM: Primary internal fixation of femoral neck fractures. *Arch Surg* 1975;110:20-26.

27. Phemister DB: The pathology of ununited fractures of the neck of the femur with special reference to the head. *J Bone Joint Surg* 1939;21:681-693.

28. Bauer DC, Cummings SR, Tao JL, et al: Hyperthyroidism increases the risk of hip fractures: A prospective study. *J Bone Miner Res* 1992;7:S121.

29. Pentecost RL, Murray RA, Brindley HH: Fatigue, insufficiency, and pathologic fractures. *JAMA* 1964;187:1001-1004.

30. Dorne HL, Lander PH: Spontaneous stress fractures of the femoral neck. *AJR* 1985;144:343-347.

31. Wright TM, Hayes WC: The fracture mechanics of fatigue crack propagation in compact bone. *J Biomed Mater Res* 1976;10:637-648.

32. Misol S, Samaan N, Ponseti IV: Growth hormone in delayed fracture union. *Clin Orthop* 1971;74:206-208.

33. Boivin G, Grousson B, Meunier PJ: X-ray microanalysis of fluoride distribution in microfracture calluses in cancellous iliac bone from osteoporotic patients treated with fluoride and untreated. *J Bone Miner Res* 1991;6:1183-1190.

34. Einhorn TA, Vigorita VJ: Unique histology of the fracture callus in a sodium fluoride (NaF)-treated osteoporotic patient with hip fracture, in Christiansen C, Johansen JS, Riis BJ (eds): *Osteoporosis. 1987/International Symposium on Osteoporosis, Alborg, Denmark*. Copenhagen, Denmark, Osteopress, 1987, pp 262-265.

35. Boden SD, Joyce ME, Oliver B, et al: Estrogen receptor in mRNA expression in callus during fracture healing in the rat. *Calcif Tissue Int* 1989;45:324-325.

36. Lucas TS, Einhorn TA: Stress fracture of the femoral neck during rehabilitation after heart transplantation. *Arch Phys Med Rehabil* 1993;74:1004-1006.

37. Kiel DP, Baron JA, Anderson JJ, et al: Smoking eliminates the protective effect of oral estrogens on the risk for hip fracture among women. *Ann Intern Med* 1992;116:716-721.

38. Chapuy MC, Arlot ME, Duboeuf F, et al: Vitamin D3 and calcium to prevent hip fractures in elderly women. *N Engl J Med* 1992;327:1637-1642.

Chapter 4

Osteoporosis in the Elderly

C. Conrad Johnston, Jr., MD
Charles W. Slemenda, DrPH

Osteoporosis may be defined as a disease characterized by low bone mass, increased skeletal fragility, and an increased incidence of fractures. Although the most important clinical consequence is fracture, an understanding of the underlying conditions that increase the incidence of fracture could lead to effective means of reducing fracture incidence.

Osteoporotic fractures occur because of fragility of the skeleton and/or trauma to the site of fracture. Although trauma resulting from falls is a leading cause of fracture, the underlying skeletal fragility makes an important contribution to fracture pathogenesis and will be discussed here.

Low bone mass at the fracture site certainly contributes to increased fracture frequency among the elderly, but other factors may also contribute as well. It has been shown that the trabeculae of cancellous bone are not simply thinned with age, but are actually lost.[1,2] Loss of horizontal connecting trabeculae leads to instability of the remaining vertical trabeculae. These architectural changes should produce fragility of the skeleton. That such changes exist is well documented, but how much they contribute quantitatively to the increased fracture frequency is not known, because such changes cannot be measured in vivo. Some evidence suggests that these changes may be important, however. In a published study by Kleerekoper and associates,[3] subjects with and without vertebral fracture were matched for age, sex, menopausal status, and some indices of bone mass. Trabecular plate density was lower in those with fracture. The presence of preexisting vertebral fractures contributes to the risk of subsequent fracture more than can be accounted for on the basis of bone mass alone;[4] this could be caused by the architectural abnormalities discussed, but other factors might be responsible as well. For example, the presence of a fracture in one region of the spine could contribute to a shift in loadbearing in the remaining vertebrae, possibly increasing the strain on the anterior edges of the remaining vertebral bodies. Kleerekoper and associates[3] have also noted that preexisting fractures elsewhere also increase the risk of spine fractures independent of bone mass. This observation is consistent with some structural property of bone contributing to fracture susceptibility, at least in the spine, where the proportion of trabecular bone is highest. Similar to the architectural changes, fatigue or microdamage is found in the skeleton and could contribute to fragility,[5] but how much such changes contribute quantitatively is unknown. In addition, when bones are tested in vitro there is a high correlation between mass and strength.[6]

Several prospective studies have shown that measurement of bone mass is a good index of risk for subsequent fracture.[7-12] Measurements of the radius, spine, heel, and lumbar spine have all demonstrated relative risks for fracture in the range of 1.5 to 2.0 per standard deviation (SD) change in bone mass. The fracture outcomes in these studies have included spine, all nonspine, and total fractures. It has also been shown that a single bone mass measurement of any of these sites can predict hip fractures.[7,10] The issue of the value of bone mass measurements at the site of fracture has been debated, but recent data have shown that relative risks for hip fracture are near 3.0 (per SD change in bone mass) when hip measurements are used for prediction.[12] The implications of this are greater than is first apparent. Whereas with a relative risk of 2.0, a person one SD below the mean has a fourfold increase in fracture risk compared to someone one SD above the mean, this rises to a ninefold difference when the relative risk is 3.0. The increase in discrimination is marked. Thus, there is ample evidence that low bone mass at the site of fracture is one of the major determinants of fracture risk.

Other skeletal characteristics may also contribute to fracture risk. It has been recently shown that femoral neck length, a measurement that can be obtained from the usual hip scans, contributes to hip fracture risk, independently of bone mass. Each one SD increase in hip axis length was associated with an almost twofold increase in hip fracture risk.[13] Although this measurement is not routinely made at present, it is possible that the manufacturers of scanning equipment could add this value to their software once normal values are established. Confirmation of this result in other samples would further strengthen its value.

Low bone mass among the elderly may be caused by low peak bone mass or excessive bone loss: at age 70, peak bone mass and loss contribute equally.[14]

Peak bone mass has a large genetic determinant. In studies of twins, from 70% to 80% of peak bone mass can be attributed to genetic factors.[15-17] However, 20% to 30% may be influenced by environmental factors, and small changes in peak bone mass within the population may make large differences in fracture rates. This is in part because some fracture rates increase exponentially,[18] and it can also be inferred from the changes in relative risk of subsequent fractures. In addition, in some published studies differences in peak bone mass as small as 6% to 7% are associated with large differences in hip fracture rates.[19]

Nutritional factors may be important in determining peak bone mass as well. Several studies have suggested that consumption of milk in childhood is associated with increased bone mass in adulthood.[20,21] This has been attributed to the calcium in milk, but could be caused by other nutritional components. In a double-blind clinical trial where one member of each young monozygotic twin pair was given a calcium supplement and the other a placebo over a three-year period, the increased calcium intake was associated with a significant increase in acquisition of bone mass.[22] Thus, calcium intake alone can contribute to peak bone mass. Other nutritional factors, such as protein intake, could be important as well. In addition, exercise was found to be important in the determination of bone mass in the children involved in this calcium supplement study.[23] Certainly, there is adequate evidence to suggest that measures can be taken to maximize peak bone mass in spite of its large genetic determination.

Peak mass may also be affected by environmental influences acting during the third decade of life. In a recently published study, both calcium and exercise were found to have positive influences on skeletal mineral growth in women in their 20s, whereas protein intake was negatively associated with changes in skeletal mass.[24] This observation of substantial (75%) growth in the 20-year-olds is controversial, as others have suggested that skeletal growth in women ceases near age 18. It is plausible that differences in environmental influences between these populations contribute to the differences in observed rates of change in bone mass. Bone loss may begin in the fourth and fifth decades of life and will contribute increasingly to the development of low bone mass and increased fracture risk as individuals age. Estrogen deficiency is a major factor in bone loss associated with menopause[25] and with periods of amenorrhea in younger women, for example, amenorrheic runners.[26] Estrogen replacement will prevent bone loss; however, when the drug is stopped, loss begins.[27] Later on, calcium deficiency may contribute to bone loss in those with insufficient intake.[28,29] Intercurrent disease, immobilization or a sedentary lifestyle, and alcohol and tobacco abuse may be important risk factors in some individuals. Men lose bone with age, and fragility fractures occur in older men, but the mechanisms responsible for bone loss in men are not well delineated. In a study of risk factors in a group of elderly male twins measured 16 years apart, tobacco and alcohol use and perhaps level of exercise were found to be important determinants of loss.[30] Importantly, although rates of bone loss were correlated between brothers, there was no strong evidence for a genetic effect on bone loss in these men. Identical, or monozygotic (MZ), pairs demonstrated correlations of about 0.6 in contrast to correlations of 0.4 in fraternal, or dizygotic (DZ), twins. This yielded an estimate of heritability of about 0.2, which was not statistically significant. Correcting for the more similar environments in MZ pairs further reduced this correlation to near 0.4, approximately equal to that of the DZ pairs, yielding a heritability estimate of zero. Thus, there remain significant correlations between brothers, but these do not differ in MZ and DZ pairs, suggesting that common environment rather than genetic influences account for the similarities in rates of bone loss. Most of the therapeutic interventions available or under study are primarily directed at prevention of bone loss. These include hormone replacement, calcitonin, and the biphosphonates.

Summary

Although trauma from falls is important in the pathogenesis of fracture among the elderly, especially hip and distal radial fractures, the increased fragility of the skeleton is also a major underlying contributing factor. Low bone mass is a primary determinant of this increased fragility. Low bone mass at the site of fracture is caused by low peak bone mass and/or accelerated bone loss. There are important determinants of low peak bone mass and accelerated bone loss that can be altered in order to reduce skeletal fragility and its associated fractures.

References

1. Parfitt AM: Trabecular bone architecture in the pathogenesis and prevention of fracture. *Am J Med* 1987;82:68-72.

2. Aaron JE, Makins NB, Sagreiya K: The microanatomy of trabecular bone loss in normal aging men and women. *Clin Orthop* 1987;215:260-271.

3. Kleerekoper M, Villanueva AR, Stanciu J, et al: The role of three-dimensional trabecular microstructure in the pathogenesis of vertebral compression fractures. *Calcif Tissue Int* 1985;37:594-597.

4. Ross PD, Davis JW, Epstein RS, et al: Pre-existing fractures and bone mass predict vertebral fracture incidence in women. *Ann Intern Med* 1991;114:919-923.

5. Frost HM: Mechanical microdamage, bone remodeling, and osteoporosis: A review, in Deluca HF, Frost HM, Jee WSS, et al (eds): *Osteoporosis: Recent Advances in Pathogenesis and Treatment*. Baltimore, MD, University Park Press, 1981.

6. Melton LJ III, Chao EYS, Lane J: Biomechanical aspects of fractures, in Riggs BL, Melton LJ III (eds): *Osteoporosis: Etiology, Diagnosis and Management*. New York, NY, Raven Press, 1988, pp 111-131.

7. Hui SL, Slemenda CW, Johnston CC Jr: Baseline measurement of bone mass predicts fracture in white women. *Ann Intern Med* 1989;111:355-361.

8. Wasnich RD, Ross PD, Heilbrun LK, et al: Prediction of postmenopausal fracture risk with use of bone mineral measurements. *Am J Obstet Gynecol* 1985;153:745-751.

9. Wasnich RD, Ross PD, Davis JW, et al: A comparison of single and multi-site BMC measurements for assessment of spine fracture probability. *J Nucl Med* 1989;30:1166-1171.

10. Cummings SR, Black DM, Nevitt MC, et al: Appendicular bone density and age predict hip fracture in women. The Study of Osteoporotic Fractures Research Group. *JAMA* 1990;263:665-668.

11. Gärdsell P, Johnell O, Nilsson BE: Predicting fractures in women by using forearm bone densitometry. *Calcif Tissue Int* 1989;44:235-242.

12. Cummings SR, Black DM, Nevitt MC, et al: Bone density at various sites for prediction of hip fractures: The Study of Osteoporotic Fractures Research Group. *Lancet* 1993;341:72-75.

13. Faulkner KG, Glüer C-C, Palermo L, et al: Geometric measurements from dual x-ray absorptiometry scans predict hip fracture. *J Bone Miner Res* 1992;7:S117.

14. Hui SL, Slemenda CW, Johnston CC Jr: The contribution of bone loss to postmenopausal osteoporosis. *Osteoporosis Int* 1990;1:30-34.

15. Smith DM, Khairi MRA, Johnston CC Jr: The loss of bone mineral with aging and its relationship to risk of fracture. *J Clin Invest* 1975;56:311-318.

16. Slemenda CW, Christian JC, Williams CJ, et al: Genetic determinants of bone mass in adult women: A reevaluation of the twin model and the potential importance of gene interaction of heritability estimates. *J Bone Miner Res* 1991;6:561-567.

17. Pocock NA, Eisman JA, Hopper JL, et al: Genetic determinants of bone mass in adults: A twin study. *J Clin Invest* 1987;80:706-710.

18. Riggs BL, Melton LJ III: Involutional osteoporosis. *N Engl J Med* 1986;314:1676-1686.

19. Matkovic V, Kostial K, Simonovic I, et al: Bone status and fracture rates in two regions of Yugoslavia. *Am J Clin Nutr* 1979;32:540-549.

20. Sandler RB, Slemenda CW, LaPorte RE, et al: Postmenopausal bone density and milk consumption in childhood and adolescence. *Am J Clin Nutr* 1985;42:270-274.

21. Halioua L, Anderson JJ: Lifetime calcium intake and physical activity habits: Independent and combined effects on the radial bone of healthy premenopausal Caucasian women. *Am J Clin Nutr* 1989;49:534-541.

22. Johnston CC Jr, Miller JZ, Slemenda CW, et al: Calcium supplementation and increases in bone mineral density in children. *N Engl J Med* 1992;327:82-87.

23. Slemenda CW, Miller JZ, Hui SL, et al: Role of physical activity in the development of skeletal mass in children. *J Bone Miner Res* 1991;6:1227-1233.

24. Recker RR, Davies KM, Hinders SM, et al: Bone gain in young adult women. *JAMA* 1992;268:2403-2408.

25. Slemenda C, Hui SL, Longcope C, et al: Sex steroids and bone mass: A study of changes about the time of menopause. *J Clin Invest* 1987;80:1261-1269.

26. Drinkwater BL, Nilson K, Chesnut CH III, et al: Bone mineral content of amenorrheic and eumenorrheic athletes. *N Engl J Med* 1984;311:277-281.

27. Lindsay R, Hart DM, Aitken JM, et al: Long-term prevention of postmenopausal osteoporosis by oestrogen: Evidence for an increased bone mass after delayed onset of oestrogen treatment. *Lancet* 1976;1:1038-1041.

28. Dawson-Hughes B, Dallal GE, Krall EA, et al: A controlled trial of the effect of calcium supplementation on bone density in postmenopausal women. *N Engl J Med* 1990;323:878-883.

29. Holbrook TL, Barrett-Connor E, Wingard DL: Dietary calcium and risk of hip fracture: 14-year prospective population study. *Lancet* 1988;2:1046-1049.

30. Slemenda CW, Christian JC, Reed T, et al: Long-term bone loss in men: Effects of genetic and environmental factors. *Ann Intern Med* 1992;117:286-291.

Section Two

Etiology: Extrinsic Factors

Chapter 5

Biomechanics of Falls and Hip Fracture in the Elderly

Wilson C. Hayes, PhD

Introduction

As measured by frequency, influence on quality of life, and economic cost, hip fractures among the elderly are an enormous and increasing public health problem. In the United States, about 250,000 such fractures occur each year, with estimated annual costs for medical and nursing services of over $7 billion.[1,2] Approximately 20% of patients with hip fracture die within a year, and 50% can no longer walk independently. About half of patients with hip fracture cannot function without help and many are admitted to nursing homes. Because hip fracture incidence rates increase exponentially with age, continued growth in the elderly population can be expected to result in a dramatic increase in the number of hip fractures.[3] If current demographic and incidence trends continue, the number of hip fractures may well double or triple by the middle of the next century.[4,5] These statistics also have important implications for the future practice of orthopaedics. In many hospitals, hip fracture patients occupy about 50% of orthopaedic beds. If the prevalence of hip fracture continues to rise as current rates indicate, it may well be that in the next decades, orthopaedists will do little else but treat patients with hip fracture. Indeed, it has been suggested that if hip fracture rates continue to rise as predicted, treatment of these fractures can potentially overwhelm the health care system. Given the ominous implications of such predictions, it is not surprising that considerable attention has focused on the causes and prevention of hip fracture.

The conventional view is that hip fractures are caused primarily by age-related bone loss, or osteoporosis. Thus, hip fracture risk is usually associated with those factors associated with age-related bone loss: advanced age, female sex, white race, thin build, low calcium intake, a sedentary lifestyle, and smoking and drinking. And yet, for several reasons, these factors tell only part of the story. In fact, case-control studies generally show considerable overlap in densities for hip fracture patients and age- and gender-matched controls.

Moreover, intervention efforts aimed at influencing bone density through the use of calcium, estrogen, and exercise have not shown consistent reductions in hip fracture incidence in elderly patients over age 70, in whom 90% of all hip fractures occur.[6]

For these reasons, it has been suggested that it is the increasing tendency of the elderly to fall and to experience falls of increased severity that explains the lack of differences in bone densities and the disappointing results with intervention trials. Melton and Riggs[7] captured this uncertainty about fracture etiology with the question, Hip fracture: Disease or accident? While the language has changed over the years to reflect the fact that many injuries are not at all accidental but can be prevented, the fundamental question remains whether hip fracture is primarily the consequence of a fall-related injury or instead the result of age-related bone loss and its concomitant increases in bone fragility. Indeed, the very definition of an age-related fracture as an osteoporotic fracture is made by noting that the fracture is associated with minimal trauma, that is, a fall from standing height or less. However, what if certain falls from standing height do not cause minimal trauma, but trauma of sufficient magnitude to cause hip fracture in the elderly every time they occur? How then should the evidence on risk factors for hip fracture be interpreted, and what are the implications for successful prevention of this growing public health problem?

The group at the Beth Israel Orthopaedic Biomechanics Laboratory in Boston has taken the position that fall severity is a potentially dominant factor in the etiology of hip fracture. Thus, defining what is meant by a high-risk fall and placing in context the relative importance of fall mechanics and bone fragility have been central thrusts of research efforts. Some of those efforts are summarized here, beginning with a general introduction to the process of fracture risk prediction. Within that framework, a falls surveillance study, which helps define a high-risk fall and provides a first-order estimate of the relative importance of fall severity and bone fragility, is discussed. Because these findings suggest a potentially dominant role for fall mechanics, several ongoing studies on the mechanics of falls from standing height are also reviewed. Based on the increasingly refined estimates of the relative importance of fall mechanics and bone fragility afforded by these efforts, the question of whether hip fracture is primarily the consequence of injury or bone loss is addressed.

Fracture Risk Prediction

In order to predict the risk of fracture of any engineering structure, it is necessary to have information on: (1) the geometry of the structure; (2) the materials from which the structure is made; and (3) the loads to which the structure is subjected. Based on that information, engineering analyses can be used to predict, under the given loading conditions, how close the structure is to failure. Alternatively, if experimental data are available on the ultimate load-carrying capacity of the structure, knowledge of the imposed loads leads directly to an estimate of fracture risk. Consider an example. If a beam supporting the ceiling is known to withstand 10,000 N (about 2,500 lb) before failure and the beam is subjected to only 1,000 N, it can be assumed that the beam will not fail and the ceiling will not collapse. However, if the beam is subjected to close to or greater than 10,000 N, there is at least a strong likelihood that the beam will fail. This approach to fracture risk prediction can be formalized by defining a fracture risk index as the ratio of the applied loads divided by the loads necessary to cause fracture. This can be written,

$$\Phi = \text{Applied Load/Fracture Load} \tag{1}$$

in which Φ is known as the fracture risk index. Equation (1) simply states that for a fracture risk index much less than 1, failure is unlikely. For a fracture risk index close to or exceeding 1, fracture is likely.

For a biological structure such as the proximal femur, estimates of the fracture risk index require information on the forces to which the proximal femur is subjected *and* information on the forces necessary to cause fracture of the proximal femur. It is important to note that the forces in both the numerator and denominator of Equation (1) should be for the same loading conditions. That is, if the risk of fracture during gait is at issue, information is needed on the maximum forces to which the hip is subjected during gait and on the forces necessary to cause fracture under those same loading conditions. If, instead, the fracture risk index for impact loading from a fall is needed, data must be available on the maximum forces applied to the hip during a fall and on the forces required to cause fracture under the same loading conditions. Put another way, it would be inappropriate (and inaccurate) to compute a fracture risk index by forming the ratio of the forces applied during gait to the forces that cause fracture of the proximal femur under fall loading conditions.

While the assessment of fracture risk requires information on both the ultimate load-carrying capacity of the femur and on the forces to which the femur is subjected, these latter forces have been largely neglected in the literature on osteoporosis. Reflecting the dominant view that age-related fractures are primarily the consequence of bone loss and increased bone fragility, researchers have focused primarily on densitometric estimates of fracture load, neglecting the intuitively obvious but largely ignored notion that the applied forces can easily dominate the fracture process. Another simple example can help make this clear. If a person falls from a great height and lands on the hip, it makes very little difference whether the femoral bone mineral density is one standard deviation below or above age- and gender-matched norms. The hip will fracture simply because the forces are well in excess of those necessary to fracture the hip of even a young, vigorous adult. The question that is then immediately raised by this approach is whether a fall from standing height represents minimal trauma, as most have suggested, or instead trauma of sufficient magnitude to fracture the hip every time such a fall occurs. To address this question, one can first examine the forces necessary to cause fracture of the proximal femur under loading conditions simulating a fall. Next, one can focus on the process of falling in an attempt to define not only what constitutes a high-risk fall (a fall that delivers high forces to the proximal femur) but also to make estimates of the forces that occur.

Hip fracture loads can be estimated by conducting failure tests of cadaveric proximal femora tested in the laboratory under controlled loading conditions. Increasingly, such experiments are being used to test the predictive accuracy of various noninvasive densitometric assessments of bone fragility. For instance, Lotz and Hayes[8] conducted an in vitro investigation of the loads and energies needed to fracture the proximal part of the femur in 12 fresh cadaveric hips under loading conditions simulating a fall to the side, with impact on the greater trochanter. The age range of the cadaveric specimens was 53 to 81 years with a mean of 69 ± 9 [SD] years. Fracture loads were a strong linear function ($R^2 = 0.93$) of a densitometric measure based on quantitative computed tomography and cross-sectional area (Fig. 1). The measured fracture loads ranged from 778 to 4,040 N (2,110 $\pm$ 1,060 [SD] N) and the work to fracture (a measure of energy absorbed during the failure process) was from 5 to 51 (26.5 $\pm$ 11). These data on fracture energy will be compared later with the energies available in falls from standing height. For the moment, however, the data on fracture load (Fig. 1) can be used in the denominator of Equation (1) to make estimates of the fracture risk index. Estimates of the applied load, however, require that how people fall be determined. A falls surveillance study designed to determine the importance of fall severity in the etiology of hip fracture will be used for this purpose.

Fall Biomechanics as Determinants of Hip Fracture Risk

Over 90% of hip fractures among the elderly are the result of a fall.[9-14] Previous research on falls and falling in the elderly has focused mostly on those host and environmental factors that result in a loss of balance and in the initiation of a fall.[11,14-24] By contrast, little is known about the mechanics of the fall itself or about the role of descent and impact in the etiology of hip fracture. Cummings and Nevitt[25] have hypothesized that four conditions must be met for a fall to cause a hip fracture: impact near the hip, failure of protective responses, insufficient energy absorption by local soft tissues, and transmission of residual force that exceeds the strength of the proximal femur. A large difference between the potential energy available in a typical fall and the comparatively low energy required to fracture

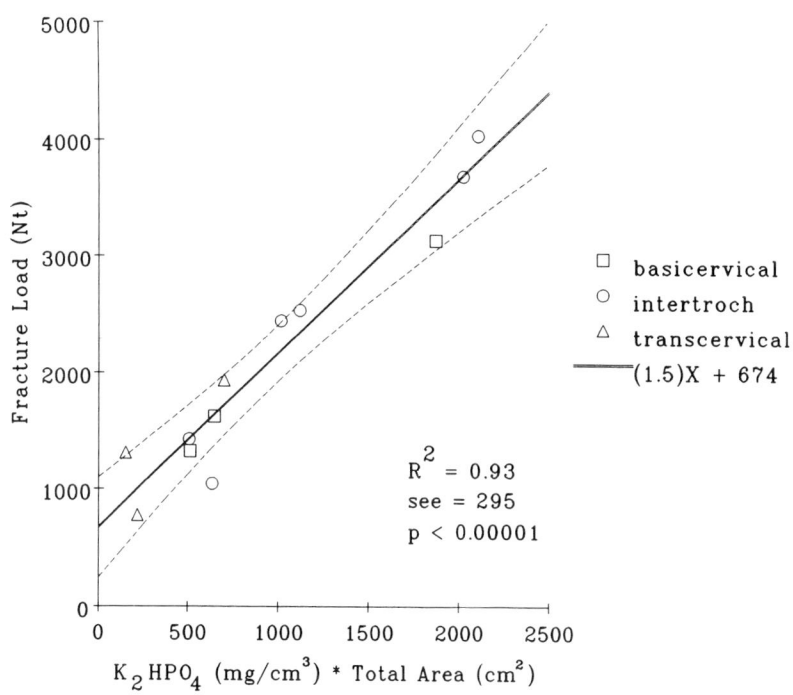

Fig. 1 *Fracture load versus average intertrochanteric equivalent mineral density as measured by quantitative computed tomography multiplied by total bone area, with symbols used for bones that failed by basicervical, intertrochanteric, or transcervical fracture. See = standard error of estimate. (Reproduced with permission from Lotz JC, Hayes WC: The use of quantitative computed tomography to estimate risk of fracture of the hip from falls. J Bone Joint Surg 1990;72A:689-700.)*

the cadaveric hip in vitro has also been noted. This difference suggests that significant energy-absorbing mechanisms must operate during those falls that do not result in fracture.[26-28] The lack of information on the position of the body at impact and on the use of strategies to absorb energy during a fall has also been noted, as has the potential role of trochanteric soft tissues in protecting against hip fracture in obese subjects.[27] However, data are not available on the potential energies available in real falls or on the typical configurations the body assumes during falling. Surprisingly, except for an anecdotal report,[29] little is known about the body sites where impact occurs for falls that do or do not result in fracture.

A surveillance effort in institutionalized elderly patients addressed some of these issues and identified aspects of the descent and impact phases of a fall that increase the risk of hip fracture.[30] Estimates of the potential energies available in these falls were compared with reported values for the energies required to fracture cadaveric hips in vitro. These data helped identify those aspects of fall mechanics associated with a high risk of hip fracture. Using this information, more effective intervention strategies can be designed for reducing the incidence of hip fracture from falls in the elderly.

Methods

Falls were sampled consecutively from two different sources: the Hebrew Rehabilitation Center for Aged (HRCA) and Beth Israel Hospital (BIH), both in Boston. The HRCA provides a life care environment at all levels of care for approximately 720 patients; the average patient age is 87 years and the female to male ratio is 3 to 1. All ambulatory residents of the HRCA aged 65 and older were eligible for the study. Computerized reports of falls and daily logs from each nursing unit were examined by a research assistant to identify fallers. A fall was defined as a sudden, unexpected descent from a standing, sitting, or horizontal position. Evidence of a fall was based on the recollection of the subject and/or a description of the fall from a witness. Unwitnessed falls in which subjects were unable to give accurate reports of their fall were excluded from the study. Also, falls that occurred over weekends and holidays were excluded if the research assistant was unable to obtain information about the fall within 24 hours. Information from the faller was used if the witness and the faller disagreed. Subjects aged 65 and older presenting at the BIH were included in the study if they had a hip fracture, if there was evidence of a fall prior to the fracture, and if they resided in a nursing home prior to being admitted to the hospital. Four subjects with possible spontaneous fractures were excluded, as were three subjects with hip fracture resulting from traffic accidents or other accidents that did not involve falling.

Falls in HRCA residents and in BIH patients were surveyed from December 30, 1986 to July 29, 1990. At the HRCA, a total of 3,012 falls occurred in 1,047 individuals during this time period. Because of the exclusion criteria previously mentioned, a total of 841 falls at the HRCA were studied: 88 falls resulted in hip fracture and 753 falls did not. The falls recorded at the BIH occurred in 409 subjects; 230 subjects (56%) fell only once during the study period, 81 subjects (20%) fell twice, and 98 subjects (24%) fell three or more times. An additional 94 falls in residents of nursing homes other than the HRCA, all of which resulted in hip fracture, were assessed at the BIH. In two of these falls, the subject fractured a second hip during the period of the study, so that the 94 falls occurred in 92 subjects. In summary, a total of 935 falls in 501 subjects were the units of analysis for this study. All subjects provided verbal informed consent for an interview, chart review, and brief examination for height and weight. This study was approved by the internal review boards of the HRCA and the BIH. No one refused participation.

Interviews with each HRCA resident who fell during the surveillance period and with any witnesses to the fall were completed by a research assistant within 24 hours of the fall. Additional information about the patient and the fall was obtained from HRCA medical records. At the BIH, interviews with patients with hip fracture and witnesses were conducted by a physical therapist within 5 days of admission. The research assistant and the physical therapist were blinded to the study hypotheses. For the 88 subjects who fell at the HRCA and were then taken to the BIH because the fall resulted in a hip fracture, interviews were conducted both by the BIH physical therapist and by the HRCA research assistant to ensure uniform ascertainment of data. The following variables were assessed for each fall: subject age, height, weight, Quetelet index (weight over height squared in units of kg/m^2), gender, mental status at the time of the fall, date and time of the fall, height of the fall, attempt by the subject to break the fall, dizziness or weakness prior to the fall, impact surface, fall direction, impact location on the body, activity and location of the subject at the time of the fall, and injuries resulting from the fall.

One of the following four categories for mental status, based on a standardized resident functional assessment performed bimonthly by HRCA primary care staff, was assigned by the interviewer to each subject at the time of the fall: normal, mild impairment, moderate impairment, or severe impairment.[31] To calculate the relative risk of fracture caused by mental impairment, the mental status scores were dichotomized to either impairment or normal. Fall height was divided into the following groups: fall in a horizontal position from a bed at home, fall in a horizontal position from a hospital bed, fall from a seated position, fall from standing height, fall from a height of one step, fall from a height of two steps, standing fall from a chair, and fall from a height greater than a chair. The fall height was then used to estimate the potential energy of the fall, which was calculated by multiplying patient mass times height of the center of gravity immediately prior to the fall times gravitational acceleration (9.8 m/s^2). The height of the center of gravity for the subject before a fall was assumed to be 0.58 times the subject's height[32] for subjects falling from a standing position. The height of the center of gravity for falls other than falls from standing height was calculated using the distance between the subject and the ground.

Attempts by the subject to break the fall were assessed by asking if the subject grabbed onto something or extended the hand in an attempt to break the fall. An inquiry was also made to ascertain whether a warning sign, such as dizziness or weakness, occurred prior to the fall. Lack of warning was included in the risk factors for hip fracture from a fall. Fall direction was divided into four categories: forward, sideways, backward, or straight down. The direction of the fall was dichotomized for calculation of relative risk into either a fall to the side or a fall in another direction. Impact location on the subject's body was recorded according to the description of the site of most severe impact by the subject or the witness. A variable describing impact on the hip or side of the leg was then derived from the impact location to be used as a risk factor for hip fracture. The activity at the time of the fall was divided into four levels: sedentary behavior (sitting or lying down), standing still, changing position (for example, going from a sitting position to a standing position), and walking. None of the fallers in nursing homes was participating in an activity more vigorous than walking.

Mean differences in continuous variables (subject height, subject weight, Quetelet index, and energy content of the fall) between falls that resulted in fracture and those that did not were compared by Student's t-test in the preliminary data analysis. Chi-square analysis was used to test the null hypothesis that there was no association between the categorical variables assessed for each fall (gender, mental impairment, fall height, not breaking the fall by grabbing onto something, not breaking the fall by extending the hand, lack of dizziness or weakness, falling to the side, impacting on the hip or the side of the leg, and walking at the time of the fall) and the presence of hip fracture. Relative risk estimates and the 95% confidence intervals were determined for each dichotomous risk factor. To check whether or not multiple fallers were biasing the relative risk results, risk ratios were also estimated for the first recorded fall using the subject rather than the fall as the unit of analysis. Because some of the risk factors could be intercorrelated, the data were also analyzed by maximum-likelihood backward elimination logistic regression in a main-effects model with hip fracture as the dichotomous outcome variable.

Results

The average age of the nursing home residents at the time of the first recorded fall was 87 ± 7 years (mean $\pm$ SD); the median age was 88 years. Of the 501 subjects, 78% were female. The mean height, weight, and Quetelet index of the subjects at the time of the fall and the potential energy content of the fall are given in Table 1 for falls that resulted in hip fracture versus those that did not. The falls resulting in hip fracture occurred in subjects with a significantly greater body height (1.58 m versus 1.51 m) and lower body weight (53.3 kg versus 56.3 kg) than in those subjects whose falls did not cause fracture. Estimated potential energies were 454 ± 145 J (SD) for those falls that resulted in hip fracture and 428 ± 142 J for those falls that did not. These energies were not significantly different.

From the frequency distributions and percentages for each categorical fall variable (Table 2), there was no difference in the gender of the faller for falls that resulted in hip fracture versus falls without hip fracture. In both the hip fracture group sampled at the BIH and the group without fracture sampled at the HRCA, approximately 80% of the falls occurred in females and 20% were in males. There were marked differences in both fall direction and impact location for falls that resulted in hip fracture compared with those that did not. Of the

Table 1 Comparison of falls resulting in hip fracture versus falls without hip fracture: weight, height, Quetelet index, and energy content

Property	Falls With Hip Fracture	Falls Without Hip Fracture	Significance (t-test)
Subject weight (kg)	53.3 (11.1)* (n = 178)	56.3(10.5) (n = 752)	<0.001
Subject height (m)	1.58 (0.08) (n = 174)	1.51 (0.08) (n = 742)	<0.001
Quetelet index (kg/m²)	21.3 (3.7) (n = 173)	24.5 (4.0) (n = 741)	<0.001
Energy content (J)	454 (145) (n = 126)	428 (142) (n = 711)	0.06

* Mean (standard deviation).

Table 2 Characteristics of falls: frequency distribution and column percentages of falls with hip fracture and falls without hip fracture

Factor		Number of Falls*	Number (%) With fracture	Number (%) Without fracture
Gender:	Female	754	145 (80)	609 (81)
	Male	181	37 (20)	144 (19)
Mental Status:	Severe	28	23 (13)	5 (<1)
	Moderate	146	67 (39)	79 (11)
	Mild	282	50 (29)	232 (31)
	Normal	467	33 (19)	434 (58)
Fall Height:	Stairs	2	1 (1)	1 (<1)
	Standing	650	109 (83)	541 (75)
	Chair	168	9 (7)	159 (22)
	Bed	30	12 (9)	18 (3)
Warning:	None	576	67 (89)	509 (74)
	Dizziness	98	7 (9)	91 (13)
	Weakness	84	1 (1)	83 (12)
	Limpness	8	0	8 (1)
Grabbed Support:	No	538	47 (83)	491 (75)
	Yes	172	10 (17)	162 (25)
Extended Arm:	No	397	46 (82)	351 (54)
	Yes	308	10 (18)	298 (46)
Fall Direction:	Sideways	190	41 (58)	149 (22)
	Forward	126	12 (17)	114 (17)
	Straight down	122	8 (11)	114 (17)
	Backward	308	10 (14)	298 (44)
Impact Location:	Hip/side of leg	84	36 (62)	48 (7)
	Front of legs	58	4 (7)	54 (8)
	Arms	69	3 (5)	66 (10)
	Buttocks	332	14 (24)	318 (47)
	Head/neck	121	1 (2)	120 (18)
	Trunk	73	0	73 (11)
Activity:	Walking	346	66 (56)	280 (39)
	Standing still	79	8 (7)	71 (10)
	Changing position	340	37 (31)	303 (42)
	Sedentary	65	6 (5)	59 (8)
	Stairs	4	1 (1)	3 (<1)

* Total number of falls = 935.

71 falls with fracture in which the fall direction was known, 41 (58%) fell to the side, whereas only 8 (11%) fell backward. By contrast, of the 675 falls without hip fracture in which the fall direction was known, 149 (22%) fell to the side and 298 (44%) fell backward. Of the 58 falls with hip fracture in which impact location was known, 36 (62%) reported impact on the hip or side of the leg and only 14 (24%) reported impact on the buttocks. Of the 679 falls without fracture, only 48 (7%) had impact on the hip or side of the leg, whereas 318 (47%) reported impact on the buttocks.

Table 3 gives the chi-square results and the relative risk estimates for the dichotomous risk variables evaluated for each fall. By this analysis, the following factors were associated with hip fracture from a fall: mental impairment, falling from standing height or higher, lack of dizziness or weakness, failure to use the arm to break the fall, falling to the side, impacting the body in the region of the hip, and walking at the time of the fall. In particular, impacting the hip or side of the leg was associated with a relative risk of 12.6 (95% confidence interval, 7.8 to 20.3). The factors that did not associate significantly with hip fracture were whether or not the subject grabbed a support and whether or not the subject was female.

When the first recorded fall for each subject was used to test the hypotheses that weight, height, Quetelet index, and energy content of the fall were equal in fallers with hip fracture versus fallers without hip fracture, the results were the same as those given in Table 1. Subjects with hip fracture were taller ($p<0.001$), lighter ($p=0.004$), and had a lower Quetelet index ($p<0.001$) than subjects without hip fracture. Using the first recorded fall, chi-square analyses of the factors listed in Table 3 showed the following to be significantly related to hip fracture: mental impairment ($p<0.001$), falling from standing height or higher ($p=0.03$), lack of warning ($p=0.003$), failure to extend the arm ($p<0.001$), falling to the side ($p<0.001$), impacting hip region ($p<0.001$), and walking ($p<0.001$).

There was a large percentage of missing data for some of the fall variables such as fall direction, impact location, and use of the extended arm (Table 3). When mental status of the subject was cross-tabulated with the presence or absence of missing data for each variable, significant associations ($p<0.001$) with missing data were found for all variables in Table 3. Approximately 30% of the responses were missing for falls in which the faller was graded as mentally impaired, whereas only about 10% were missing in falls where the mental status was designated as normal. Therefore, the relationships between hip fracture after falling and the characteristics of the fall were investigated further by controlling for mental impairment with the use of Cochran-Mantel-Haenszel (CMH) statistics. The characteristics that showed a significant general association with hip fracture by the CMH statistic were the same as those in Table 3, except for falling from standing height or higher ($p=0.06$). The CMH statistics adjusted relative risk estimates with mental impairment as a con-

Table 3 Relative risk estimates for dichotomous variables

Risk Factor	Relative Risk	95% Confidence Interval	Significance (Chi-square)	Number (%) of Missing Data
Female	0.9	0.7–1.3	0.7	0 (0%)
Mental impairment	4.3	3.0–6.2	<0.001	12 (1%)
Standing height or higher	1.6	1.0–2.5	0.03	85 (9%)
No dizziness/ weakness	2.8	1.4–5.6	0.003	169 (18%)
Lack of grabbing support	1.5	0.8–2.9	0.2	225 (24%)
Lack of extending arm	3.6	1.8–7.0	<0.001	230 (25%)
Falling to the side	4.0	2.6–6.2	<0.001	189 (20%)
Impacting hip region	12.6	7.8–20.3	<0.001	198 (21%)
Walking	1.8	1.3–2.5	<0.001	95 (10%)

founding variable remained within the 95% confidence intervals given in Table 3 and the test for homogeneity of relative risk ratios was not rejected for each variable, indicating that mental impairment was not confounding the associations.

Independent variables associated with the occurrence of a hip fracture during a fall by the logistic regression model are shown in Table 4. Only 609 out of 935 falls were used in the multiple regression because of the large number of missing values for some of the effect variables. Associations of hip fracture with impact location on the hip, failure to use the outstretched hand during the fall, and lack of dizziness or weakness immediately prior to the fall, were all significant in the multiple regression. The odds ratio for having a hip fracture given that impact was on the hip or side of the leg was 35 (95% confidence interval, 11.7−104.7) after adjusting for the linear effects of the other variables in the model. Low Quetelet index and low energy content of the fall were also found to be independent predictors of hip fracture. The univariate associations of hip fracture with mental impairment, falling from standing height or higher, falling to the side, and walking at the time of the fall (Table 3) did not result in significant associations in the multiple regression.

Discussion

These results suggest that the risk of hip fracture from falls among nursing home residents is in large part a function of impact site and fall direction, the potential energy of the fall, and the use of active and passive energy absorption mechanisms such as extending the hand to break the fall and the deformation of soft tissues at the site of impact. Six factors were identified by logistic regression to predict hip fracture after a fall: impact location on the body, energy content

Table 4 Results of multiple logistic regression with hip fracture as the outcome

Factor	Coefficient (Standard Error)	Adjusted Odds Ratio	95% Confidence Interval for Odds Ratio
Impacting hip region	3.55 (0.56)	35.0	11.7 – 104.7
Lack of extending arm	1.75 (0.57)	5.8	1.9 – 17.7
Female	1.60 (0.75)	4.9	1.1 – 21.5
No dizziness/weakness	1.53 (0.71)	4.6	1.1 – 18.6
Quetelet index	−0.63 (0.11)		
Energy content	0.014 (0.004)		

of the fall, failure to extend the arm, Quetelet index, lack of dizziness or weakness, and the gender of the faller. Impacting on the hip or side of the leg appears to be the most important determinant of hip fracture risk among fallers who are nursing home residents, raising the risk over tenfold.

This study has several strengths: all subjects were recruited consecutively from two well-defined institutionalized samples (ambulatory residents at the HRCA and hip fracture patients admitted to the BIH) and were interviewed within 5 days after the fall, which is sooner than in previous studies. In addition, the falls surveillance instrument, adapted and expanded from an instrument used by Nevitt and associates,[22] also included new questions on the mechanics of the fall. Therefore, certain falls (those to the side, with impact on the hip or side of the leg) were identified as presenting a high risk of hip fracture. As such, the data extend previous falls·surveillance studies that focused primarily on why subjects fall with information on the importance of how subjects fall in the etiology of hip fracture. Finally, analysis controlling for missing data validated the hypotheses.

This study also has several important limitations; most importantly, the use of self-reported data from elderly subjects (average age 87 years) who had just experienced a life-threatening, traumatic event. The inability of elderly fallers to describe the circumstances of their fall or even to recall that a fall has occurred within three months prior to contact is well known.[33] Therefore, information about which the subjects were uncertain was recorded as unknown. This attempt to be rigorous about excluding uncertain responses accounts for the high percentage of missing values, particularly for those variables related to the mechanics of the fall. Steps were taken to ensure that the interviewers at both the HRCA and the BIH were blinded to the hypotheses guiding the study. There was concern, particularly among fallers who fractured their hip, that subjects would bias their responses on fall direction and impact site because of pain at the affected hip. However, it should also be noted that hip fracture patients rarely report pain overlying the greater trochanter but instead describe pain referred to the inguinal region.

A second limitation is that the study was conducted on nursing home residents and therefore does not identify factors that are associated with hip fracture from falls in community-based elderly subjects. Nursing home residents are frail and do not participate in strenuous activities, as indicated by assessment of activity at the onset of the fall. Several characteristics may be enhanced in a nursing home sample (compared with community dwellers) such as delayed reaction times, reduced lower extremity strength, and slow gait, which would increase the likelihood of falling to the side and impacting on the hip or side of the leg.[25] As a result, other factors that were not significant in this study or were not assessed could prove to be important factors in the etiology of hip fractures outside of the nursing home.

It is generally assumed that the increasing incidence of hip fracture in the elderly is the result of a combination of age-related factors including increased risk of falling, changes in neuromuscular function, and osteoporosis.[25,27] There was no direct measure of the bone mineral density of the proximal femur or of the energy-absorbing capacity of the soft tissues overlying the hip, so the effects of these factors could not be examined directly. The gender of the faller did not result in a significant association with fracture when it was considered alone, yet it became a significant predicting variable when adjustments were made for the effects of the other independent variables. This result suggests that such gender-associated factors as bone density and hormonal differences may become important in determining hip fracture from a fall if the impact site, the available potential energy, and the body habitus are taken into account.

On the other hand, a comparison of the potential energies associated with falls in this population of elderly nursing home residents with the energies required to fracture the elderly cadaveric hip in vitro would indicate that factors related to the mechanics of the fall are more important than those related to bone fragility. As previously noted, Lotz and Hayes[8] recently reported data on the fracture loads and energies for cadaveric proximal femora (patient age range, 53 to 81 years; mean 69 ± 9 years) loaded so as to simulate a fall with direct impact on the lateral greater trochanter. Fracture energies ranged from 5 to 51 J (mean and SD, 26.5 ± 11 J). By contrast, the potential energies associated with falls among these elderly nursing home residents were 454 ± 145 J for falls resulting in fracture and 428 ± 142 J for falls without fracture. These energy values are nearly an order of magnitude greater than the maximum in vitro fracture energy and more than 15 times the average in vitro fracture energy.

These data on potential energies associated with falls thus confirm earlier suggestions[13,28] that much less energy is needed to fracture the proximal femur than is available even in simple falls from standing height (which represented over 75% of all falls reported). These findings also suggest that a fall from standing height should no longer be considered as representing minimal trauma and used as a way to define a fracture of the hip as an osteoporotic fracture. The data presented here instead suggest that a fall from standing height, especially if associated with direct impact on the hip or side of the leg, is associated with sufficient potential energy to cause fracture in every instance. Furthermore, because a fracture of the hip occurs in fewer than 5% of falls in nursing home residents, the data suggest that substantial energy must usually be absorbed by the deformation of trochanteric or gluteal soft tissues, eccentric contraction of the leg muscles to slow the descent, and the use of the outstretched arm to break the fall.

The potentially dominant confounding role of fall severity is a likely explanation for the failure of most densitometric studies to distinguish clearly between hip fracture patients and age- and gender-matched controls, especially in the elderly population over age 70 in whom over 90% of hip fractures occur.[34] The importance of fall severity may also help to explain the generally disappointing results with intervention efforts directed toward the maintenance of bone strength in this population.[6] More precise determinations of the relative risks associated with fall mechanics, body habitus, and bone fragility will require simultaneous characterization of these factors. From the data reported here for elderly nursing home residents, however, the most important determinant of hip fracture risk among elderly fallers is probably whether or not impact occurs directly on the hip or side of the leg, followed by measures of the potential energy available in the fall and an index of obesity. Densitometric measures of bone fragility would be expected to exert a moderate role in hip fracture etiology among elderly fallers and to be significant only after accounting for the confounding effects of fall severity and body habitus. If these hypotheses prove correct, the findings would have important implications for the design of interventions against hip fracture in elderly populations.

Energy Estimates for Experimental Falls From Standing Height

These fall surveillance data indicate that falls to the side with impact directly on the greater trochanter are particularly dangerous, raising the risk of hip fracture over 30-fold. Moreover, the energies available in falls from standing height are more than an order of magnitude greater than the energies required to fracture the elderly cadaveric hip under loading conditions meant to simulate a fall. Given that the available energy in a fall is so much greater than that required to fracture the elderly femur, the question naturally arises as to why the hip does not fracture every time a fall occurs. Because less than 5% of falls actually result in a hip fracture, a number of mechanisms must be at work to reduce the injury potential of those falls. One obvious mechanism suggested by the fall surveillance studies is that most falls must not be to the side or involve impact directly on the hip. A second mechanism is that some of the available potential energy could be absorbed during the descent phase. To address this issue, van den Kroonenberg and associates[35] used high-speed video of experimental falls by young adult volunteers to analyze the impact velocities and body configurations during experimental falls from standing height. They addressed the following questions: (1) What are the ranges of hip impact velocities and energies associated with sideways falls from standing height? (2) What are typical body configurations at impact? and (3) How do protective reflexes such as muscle activation or using the outstretched hand influence these variables?

The subjects were all college athletes (three males and three females, ranging in age from 19 to 26). The falls were initiated by the subjects based on instructions to launch themselves sideways and subsequently fall as naturally as possible before landing on a 10 inch-thick foam mattress. Several categories of falls were investigated: (1) muscle-active versus muscle-relaxed fall; (2) falling from a standing position or while walking; and (3) falls in which the outstretched arm was used to break the fall. Surface electromyograms were used as a qualitative indicator of the muscle activity of the quadriceps and hamstrings. Each fall was videotaped (Fig. 2) at 60 frames/s so that the trajectory of a marker placed on the left hip could be digitized. The resulting displacement versus time curves were fit by polynomials and the hip impact velocity was calculated by differentiation. Estimates of the velocities that would have occurred had the subjects impacted on the floor (instead of the mattress) were also obtained. Data were analyzed using a two-factor, repeated measures analysis of variance with muscle-active versus muscle-relaxed and walking versus standing as trial factors. The potential energy available in the fall was correlated with the average hip impact velocity for each subject.

There were no significant differences in impact velocities or body configurations for male versus female fallers or for falls initiated from walking or standing. For the six subjects, hip impact velocities at the mattress range from 1.95 to 3.70 m/s (2.75 ± 0.451 [SD]). Estimated impact velocities at the floor range from 2.14 to 4.25 m/s (3.19 ± 0.45 m/s). Surprisingly, muscle-relaxed falls resulted in a 7% decrease in estimated impact velocity at the floor compared to muscle-active falls (3.31 ± 0.39 versus 3.09 ± 0.41 m/s; $p=0.038$). Available potential energy was a poor predictor of hip impact velocity ($p=0.8$). Finally, despite the instruction to break the fall with the arm or hand, only two of the six subjects were able to do so. In the remaining subjects, hip impact occurred first, followed by contact with the arm or hand.

These data, the first available on impact velocities and energies for simulated falls from standing height, shed additional light on the etiology of hip fracture. Rather than the 10- to 20-fold difference between available potential energy and the energy required to fracture the proximal femur, these simulated falls suggest differences closer to between 2- and 10-fold. The data thus indicate that substantial en-

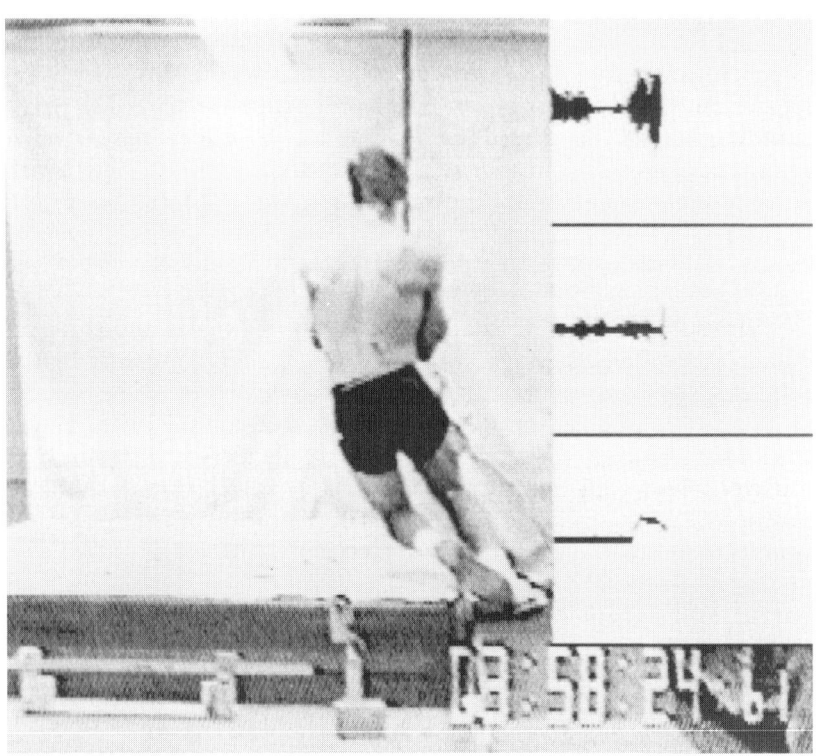

Fig. 2 *Video frame from an experimental fall in a young adult volunteer. Falls were used to estimate body configurations, velocities and kinetic energies at impact. Impact with the floor was prevented using a 10 inch-thick foam mattress. Several categories of falls were investigated: (1) muscle-active versus muscle-relaxed; (2) falling from a standing position or from walking; and (3) falls in which the outstretched arm was used to break the fall. Surface electromyogram (EMG) was used as a qualitative indicator of neuromuscular activity of the quadriceps (top window) and hamstrings (middle window). Force plate data are seen in the bottom window.*

ergy is absorbed during the descent phase by eccentric contraction of the lower extremity musculature and by residual stiffness of the knee and hip. While these falls were not unintentional and did not occur in the elderly, the calculated floor impact energies, ranging from 63 to 248 J, are believed to be considerably more accurate than previous estimates based on simple energy conservation. Noting that the average fracture energies for elderly cadaveric femora were 26.5 J,[8] these energies are from 2.4- to 9.4-fold greater than is required to fracture the hip. The surprising reductions in impact velocities found in muscle-relaxed falls appear to be the consequence of hip impact occurring closer to the feet in the muscle-relaxed case. This finding provides yet another mechanism whereby falling relaxed reduces the injury potential of a fall. The fact that these young, athletic volunteers in most cases could not, despite instructions, use the outstretched arm to break a sideways fall confirms the observations of Holliday and associates[36] from videotapes of unintentional falls among elderly nursing home residents. In almost all cases, elderly fallers attempted to use the outstretched arm to break the fall but were unable to prevent the hip or buttock from impacting the floor first. Especially for sideways falls, the body configuration at impact may simply preclude effective use of the outstretched arm to break the fall.

Prediction of Fall Impact Forces

Knowledge of the kinetic energy at impact can be used to estimate the force applied to the hip during a sideways fall with impact on the greater trochanter. The simplest approach to such a prediction is through use of the impulse-momentum principle from physics. Assuming that the hip impact force F is constant and acts over a time period Δt, the impulse-momentum principle may be written:

$$F\Delta t = m(v_2 - v_1) \tag{2}$$

in which m is the effective mass of the body at impact, v_2 is the velocity of the body after impact, and v_1 is the velocity of the body just prior to impact. The effective mass is defined as that fraction of body mass that actually participates in the impact event (if the extremities are free to move with respect to the trunk at impact, their mass may not play a role at impact, thus reducing the effective mass). If post-impact velocity is assumed to be equal and opposite to the preimpact velocity (the subject is assumed to bounce slightly at impact), Equation (2) can be rewritten as:

$$F = 2mv/\Delta t \tag{3}$$

in which v is now the impact velocity. Using the average floor impact velocities determined by van den Kroonenberg and associates,[35] the effective mass of a typical elderly female, and an impact time of 60 milliseconds, the predicted hip impact force is about 3000 N, a value that is 50% greater than the average force required to fracture the elderly cadaveric hip in vitro.

Such force estimates are obviously crude and depend on a series of assumptions about which there is considerable uncertainty. To improve these estimates of hip impact force, Robinovitch and associates[37] developed a simple experiment (the pelvis release experiment) that allowed prediction of potentially injurious fall impact forces. In addition to providing the estimated force and rate of loading to the impacted hip in a fall, these pelvis release experiments addressed the following question: How are fall impact forces influenced when the body contacts the ground in a state of muscle relaxation as opposed to muscle contraction? To address this question, Robinovitch and associates[37] tested human volunteers and examined the differences in impact response arising when subjects were encouraged to contract the trunk muscles. Finally, to evaluate the risk of hip fracture in a fall resulting in direct lateral impact to the hip, they compared pelvis release predictions of full impact force with previous measures of the force required to fracture the proximal femur in vitro under load conditions simulating a fall.

Seven males and seven females ranging in age from 20 to 35 years and in body weight from 489 to 916 N participated in the study. To perform a pelvis release experiment, each subject lay with the lateral aspect of the greater trochanter contacting a high-fidelity force plate, the lower leg and shoulder resting on platforms, and the pelvis cradled in a canvas sling (Fig. 3). Before the test, the pelvis of the subject was raised slightly and then released. The resulting oscillatory force versus time record was fit with a mass-spring-damper model and used to determine the effective mass of the body at impact and the spring stiffness k and the damping factor b of the soft tissues overlying the greater trochanter. Just prior to the experiment, the subject was instructed either to completely relax the body (muscle-relaxed) or to contract the trunk and back muscles in an attempt to raise the head and shoulder off the shoulder support (muscle-active). Muscle activity was monitored in all trials through electromyographic surface electrodes placed on the spinalis portion of the erector spinae muscle at the level of the tenth rib, the posterior superior portion of the external oblique, and the gluteus medius 5 cm superior to the greater trochanter.

Force versus time records for a typical male subject (Fig. 4) demonstrate that erector spinae electromyogram increased considerably in the muscle-active case. Furthermore, the impact force increased from approximately 180 N in the muscle-relaxed case to 260 N in the muscle-active case. Furthermore, based on the mass-spring-dashpot model, muscle contraction caused significant increases in the effective mass m (an increase of 58% from 31 to 49 kg). In order to estimate the typical force applied to the proximal femur for falls in both muscle-relaxed and muscle-active states, average values of the effective mass m and the values of the trochanteric soft-tissue stiffness and damping were incorporated into equations describing the dynamics of impact, with velocity given by a free-fall of the effective mass from an initial height of 0.7 m. For men, the effective mass averaged 39 kg in the muscle-relaxed state and 49 kg in the muscle-active state, values that represent 50% and 63% of the average whole body mass, respectively. In women, the effective mass averaged 31 kg in the muscle-relaxed state and 37.6 kg in the muscle-active state, representing 50% and 60% of average whole body mass, respectively. The predicted peak forces as a function of fall height demonstrate a dramatic increase in peak force for the muscle-active state in men, but not in women (Fig. 5). At a fall height of 0.7 meters (a reasonable average value for a fall from standing height), the peak force in males

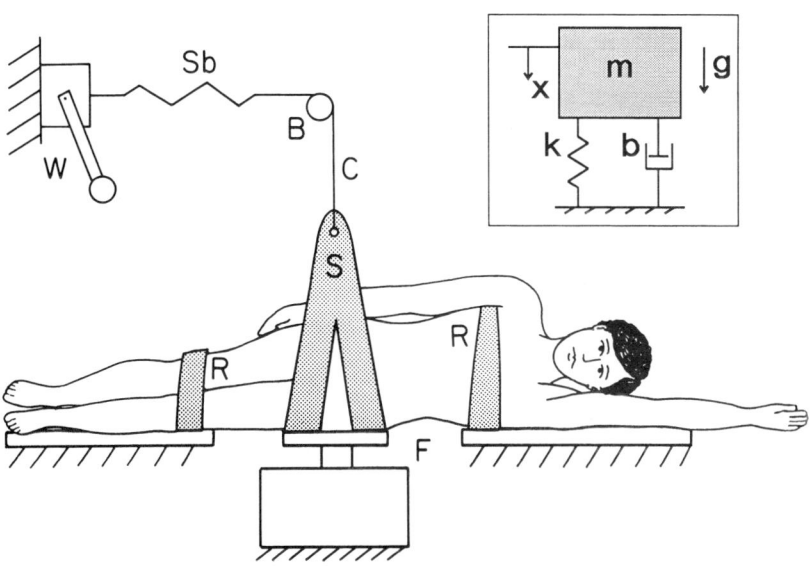

Fig. 3 *Apparatus for pelvis release experiments. F, high fidelity force platform; S, pelvis holding sling; R, shoulder and knee restraints; C, steel chain; B, electromagnetic brake; Sb, bias spring; W, winch. The mass-spring-damper model used to simulate the impact response of the body in pelvis release experiments is shown in the inset. (Reproduced with permission from Robinovitch SN, Hayes WC, McMahon TA: Prediction of femoral impact forces in falls on the hip. J Biomech Eng 1991;113:366-374.)*

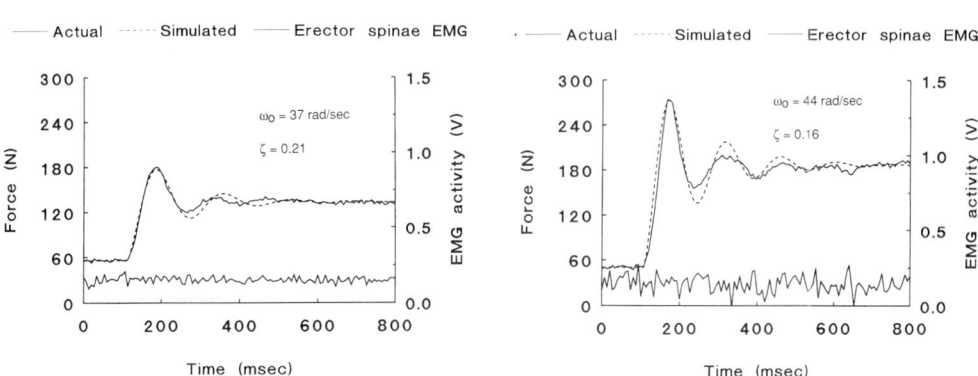

Fig. 4 *Results of two pelvis release experiments showing the effects of muscle contraction on the observed response: **left**, male subject in muscle-relaxed measure; **right**, male subject in muscle-active measure. The solid curves give measured results; the broken curves show the predictions of a simple mathematical model. (Reproduced with permission from Robinovitch SN, Hayes WC, McMahon TA: Prediction of femoral impact forces in falls on the hip. J Biomech Eng 1991:113:366-374.)*

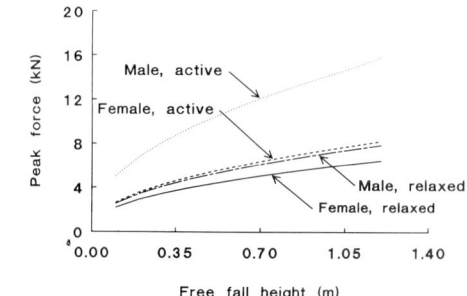

Fig. 5 *Effect of drop height, gender, and muscle activity on predicted peak impact force. Peak forces were higher in men than women, and higher in the muscle-active than muscle-relaxed state (with a pronounced difference in men but not in women). (Reproduced with permission from Robinovitch SN, Hayes WC, McMahon TA: Prediction of femoral impact forces in falls on the hip. J Biomech Eng 1991;113:366-374.)*

in the muscle-relaxed state was 6,100 N and 12,100 N in the muscle-active state. Corresponding values for women were 5,050 N and 6,370 N, respectively. Note that these values can be used in Equation (1) to estimate the fracture risk index. For a woman, falling in the muscle-relaxed condition, the estimated fracture risk index for a fall from standing height with impact directly on the greater trochanter is about 2.7. For a man, depending on whether the fall is in a muscle-relaxed or muscle-active state, the fracture risk index ranges from 2.9 to 5.7, respectively.

These results suggest that the state of muscle activity at impact is an important determinant of fall fracture risk. For example, muscle activation in males caused 100% increases in predicted average peak force. These changes reflected two phenomena caused by contraction of the trunk muscles at impact: (1) an increase in the effective mass m as more of the trunk and lower extremities played a role at impact; and (2) an increase in the rigidity of muscular connections between the trunk, pelvis, and lower limbs. Therefore, while neuro-muscular control in the descent phase of the fall may reduce the velocity of impact and allow the faller to adjust the body into a safe landing configuration, striking the ground in a stiff state actually increases the impact force. These findings also confirm the well-established notion that falling in a relaxed state reduces the potential for injury.

In order to compare the fall impact force predictions of this study with the measured in vitro fracture strength of the proximal femur, consider an average individual falling from a height of 0.7 m and landing in a position duplicating the body configuration of the pelvis release experiments. Taking an average of the values obtained for younger men and women, peak hip impact forces of approximately 5,600 N are predicted for the muscle-relaxed state, and 8,600 N for the muscle-active state. These values are significantly greater than the measured in vitro fracture forces measured by Lotz and Hayes.[8] Using the average values of the in vitro fracture forces (2,110 N) and the average estimated hip impact force for a relaxed fall from the pelvis release experiments of Robinovitch and associates[37] would indicate a fracture risk index of 2.65. That is, the forces applied to the hip during such a fall are between two and three times the forces necessary to fracture the hip under the same loading conditions. Falling in a muscle-active state raises the fracture risk index to greater than 4. Given these values, it is therefore not surprising that a fall to the side with direct impact on the greater trochanter has such a high risk of fracture.

Summary: Is Hip Fracture a Disease or an Injury?

Hip fracture is clearly a public health problem of national importance and one that may influence the future of orthopaedics in a dramatic way. Given that recent efforts directed toward the prevention of hip fracture (through the use of osteodynamic agents to ameliorate or reverse bone loss or interventions directed toward fall prevention) have not achieved consistent success in the elderly over age 70 in whom most hip fractures occur, studies have been directed toward a better understanding of fracture etiology and the design of more effective prevention strategies. The fundamental engineering principle that fracture risk is defined as the ratio of the applied loads to the fracture loads, a ratio which can be called the fracture risk index, Φ, was used to address these issues. When Φ is low, fracture is unlikely; when Φ is greater than 1, fracture can be expected. This simple paradigm focuses on two aspects of the etiology of hip fracture: (1) the forces associated with falls from standing height (which in turn cause over 90% of hip fractures); and (2) those factors associated with bone fragility. Previous research into the etiology and prevention of age-related fractures has focused nearly exclusively on osteoporosis and bone fragility, to the exclusion of the important, and potentially dominant, factors related to impact forces from falls.

The work summarized here is thus an attempt to address a series of research questions related to refining the estimates of the factor of risk for hip fracture from falls from standing height. To define the denominator of the factor of risk, the ranges of forces and energies required to fracture the elderly cadaveric hip in vitro need to be determined. From the data reported by Lotz and Hayes,[8] (Fig. 1) the average forces are about 2,100 N and the average energies are about 26.5 J. In order to provide first-order estimates of the energies available in falls from standing height in typical elderly fallers, a large falls surveillance effort was conducted, which indicated that average energies available in falls are about 440 J, or about 16 times the energy required to fracture the elderly cadaveric hip. Moreover, these falls surveillance efforts defined a high-risk fall as any fall to the side, particularly if such a fall involves direct impact on the greater trochanter. Such a fall (to the side with impact on the greater trochanter) raises the risk of fracture nearly 30-fold.

In order to provide improved estimates of the actual impact velocities and energies associated with real falls, experimental falls were conducted among young adult volunteers. These experiments suggest that many falls actually have impact energies that are somewhat less than those predicted from energy conservation principles. This reduction was probably caused by inadvertent eccentric contractions of the lower extremity musculature. The energies just prior to impact in these experimental sideways falls ranged from approximately 60 to 250 J, substantially less than the approximately 500 J of potential energy that is available prior to the descent phase of the fall. While these more precise estimates of impact energies are useful to provide first-order approximations of impact forces, improved estimates for the forces can be obtained by simulated, noninjurious falls in which the impact forces are actually measured at low load and, based on simple engineering models, used to extrapolate to the impact forces that would occur in falls from standing height. The pelvis-release experiments were performed in order to estimate the impact forces that occur in falls to the side and to determine how these forces are influenced by muscle activity at the time of impact. In females, the predicted impact forces were approximately 6,000 N and were relatively insensitive to the state of muscle contraction at impact. By contrast, the estimated impact forces in males were highly sensitive to the state of muscle contraction, ranging from about 6,000 N in the muscle-relaxed state up to about 12,000 N in the muscle-active state.

Finally, based on these estimates of the forces and energies associated with falls from standing height and on measured values for the strengths of the elderly proximal femur, how these forces and energies compare to hip fracture forces and energies actually measured in vitro in human cadaveric specimens can be determined. Based on the energies estimated from the experimental falls, the energies available at impact are about twofold to tenfold greater than the energies required to fracture the elderly cadaveric hip in vitro. More precise comparisons using forces can be obtained based on the factor of risk. Using the pelvis-release experiments to estimate the applied force, the factor of risk for a fall from standing height with impact on the greater trochanter is about 2.7 in women and, depending on the state of muscle activity at impact, ranges from about 3 to 6 in men.

These high factors of risk would suggest that a fall to the side with impact on the greater trochanter represents a very high risk of fracture in the elderly. Indeed, these risk estimates are supported by the surveillance studies, which suggest that such falls raise the risk of fracture over 30-fold.[30] At the very least, these data indicate that a fall from standing height should no longer be considered as representing minimal trauma and used to define an age-related fracture as osteoporotic. Instead, if such a fall is to the side and involves impact on the hip, the data suggest that such falls should cause fracture every time they occur. However, epidemiologic evidence indicates that less than 5% of all falls result in hip fracture.[16,22] The inescapable conclusion, then, is that most falls are not of this high-risk type. In addition, some of the energy available in a fall can be absorbed by the muscles of the lower extremity during the descent phase[35] or by use of the outstretched arm to break the fall.[30] Thus, differences in the indices of fall severity (falling to the side, landing on the hip, and failure to use the outstretched arm to break the fall or the leg muscles to slow the descent) are, along with age-related reductions in bone density, important determinants of hip fracture risk. And finally, at impact, the trochanteric soft tissues can also absorb energy, further reducing the applied load.[30,37]

These conclusions on the etiology of hip fracture also have implications for the design and implementation of hip fracture prevention efforts. Because fall impact forces appear to exceed the strength of the femur in an elderly patient by a factor of 2 or 3, it is unlikely that sufficient protection can be afforded by the use of osteodynamic agents, especially in this elderly population in whom bone density is already well below clinically recommended fracture thresholds. Especially because fall prevention efforts have proved to be disappointing,[6,38] it seems likely that more productive intervention strategies would involve attempts to reduce the severity of those falls that do occur. Such reductions in fall severity can be accomplished either through passive energy absorption strategies, through the use of trochanteric padding or energy-absorbing floors, or through exercise programs directed toward increasing lower extremity strength and keeping neuromuscular response mechanisms intact.[39] Indeed, preliminary results with trochanteric padding systems[40-43] suggest these to be a productive strategy to pursue. Moreover, data indicate that such trochanteric padding systems can be designed so that impact forces are reduced to levels below the fracture threshold for elderly cadaveric femora.[38,44] Based on such approaches and an improved understanding of the complex interplay between fall biomechanics and bone fragility in the etiology of hip fracture, there is hope that the rising epidemic of hip fractures among the elderly can be substantially reduced.

References

1. Holbrook TL, Grazier KL, Kelsey JL, et al: *The frequency of occurrence, impact, and cost of selected musculoskeletal conditions in the United States.* Presented at the Thirty-Third Annual Meeting of the American Academy of Orthopaedic Surgeons, Chicago, IL, 1984.

2. Phillips S, Fox N, Jacobs J, et al: The direct medical costs of osteoporosis for American women aged 45 and older; 1986. *Bone* 1988;9:271-279.

3. Melton LJ III, O'Fallon WM, Riggs BL: Secular trends in the incidence of hip fractures. *Calcif Tissue Int* 1987;41:57-64.

4. Cummings SR: Epidemiology of hip fractures, in Jensen J, Riis B, Christiansen C (eds): *Osteoporosis: Proceeding of the International Symposium on Osteoporosis.* Viborg, Denmark, Norhaven A/S, 1987, pp 40-43.

5. Kelsey JL, Hoffman S: Risk factors for hip fracture (editorial). *N Engl J Med* 1987;316:404-406.

6. Resnick NM, Greenspan SL: "Senile" osteoporosis reconsidered. *JAMA* 1989;261:1025-1029.

7. Melton LJ III, Riggs BL: Hip fracture: A disease and an accident, in Uhthoff HK, Stahl E (eds): *Current Concepts Bone Fragility.* Berlin, Germany, Springer-Verlag, 1986, pp 385-389.

8. Lotz JC, Hayes WC: The use of quantitative computed tomography to estimate risk of fracture of the hip from falls. *J Bone Joint Surg Am* 1990;72A:689-700.

9. Alffram PA: An epidemiologic study of cervical and trochanteric fractures of the femur in an urban population: Analysis of 1,664 cases with special reference to etiologic factors. *Acta Orthop Scand Suppl* 1964;65:9-114.

10. Backman S: The proximal end of the femur. *Acta Radiol Suppl* 1957;146:7-166.

11. Waller JA: Falls among the elderly-human and environmental factors. *Accid Anal Prev* 1978;10:21-33.

12. Hedlund R, Lindgren U: Trauma type, age, and gender as determinants of hip fracture. *J Orthop Res* 1987;5:242-246.

13. Melton LJ, Chao EYS, Lane J: Biomechanical aspects of fractures, in Riggs BL, Melton LJ III (eds): *Osteoporosis: Etiology, Diagnosis and Management.* New York, NY, Raven Press, 1988, chap 4, pp 111-131.

14. Grisso JA, Kelsey JL, Strom BL, et al: Risk factors for falls as a cause of hip fracture in women: The Northeast Hip Fracture Study Group. *N Engl J Med* 1991;324:1326-1331.

15. Ray WA, Griffin MR, Schaffner W, et al: Psychotropic drug use and the risk of hip fracture. *N Engl J Med* 1987;316:363-369.

16. Tinetti ME, Speechley M, Ginter SF: Risk factors for falls among elderly persons living in the community. *N Engl J Med* 1988;319:1701-1707.

17. Tinetti ME, Williams TF, Mayewski R: Fall risk index for elderly patients based on number of chronic disabilities. *Am J Med* 1986;80:429-434.

18. Campbell AJ, Borrie MJ, Spears GF: Risk factors for falls in a community-based prospective study of people 70 years and older. *J Gerontol* 1989;44:M112-M117.

19. Prudham D, Evans JG: Factors associated with falls in the elderly: A community study. *Age Ageing* 1981;10:141-146.

20. DeVito CA, Lambert DA, Sattin RW, et al: Fall injuries among the elderly: Community-based surveillance. *J Am Geriatr Soc* 1988;36:1029-1035.

21. Robbins AS, Rubenstein LZ, Josephson KR, et al: Predictors of falls among elderly people: Results of two-population-based studies. *Arch Intern Med* 1989;149:1628-1633.

22. Nevitt MC, Cummings SR, Kidd S, et al: Risk factors for recurrent nonsyncopal falls: A prospective study. *JAMA* 1989;261:2663-2668.

23. Lipsitz LA, Pluchino FC, Wei JY, et al: Syncope in institutionalized elderly: The impact of multiple pathological conditions and situational stress. *J Chron Dis* 1986;39:619-630.

24. Lipsitz LA, Jonsson PV, Kelly MM, et al: Causes and correlates of recurrent falls in ambulatory frail elderly. *J Gerontol* 1991;46:M114-M122.

25. Cummings SR, Nevitt MC: A hypothesis: The causes of hip fractures. *J Gerontol* 1989;44:M107-M111.

26. Muckle DS, Bentley G, Deane G, et al: Basic sciences of the hip, in Muckle DS (ed): *Femoral Neck Fractures and Hip Joint Injuries*. New York, NY, John Wiley and Sons, 1977, chap 1, pp 1-54.

27. Melton LJ III, Riggs BL: Risk factors for injury after a fall. *Clin Geriatr Med* 1985;1:525-539.

28. Frankel VH, Burstein AH: *Orthopedic Biomechanics*. Philadelphia, PA, Lea & Febiger, 1970.

29. Peck WA: Falls and hip fracture in the elderly. *Hosp Pract (Off Ed)* 1986;21:72A-72L.

30. Hayes WC, Myers ER, Morris JN, et al: Impact near the hip dominates fracture risk in elderly nursing home residents who fall. *Calcif Tissue Int* 1993;52:192-198.

31. Besdine RW: The educational utility of comprehensive functional assessment in the elderly. *J Am Geriatr Soc* 1983;31:651-656.

32. Khodadadeh S, Whittle MW, Bremble GR: Height of centre of body mass during osteoarthritic gait. *Clin Biomech* 1986;1:77-80.

33. Cummings SR, Nevitt MC, Kidd S: Forgetting falls: The limited accuracy of recall of falls in the elderly. *J Am Geriatr Soc* 1988;36:613-616.

34. Cummings SR, Kelsey JL, Nevitt MC, et al: Epidemiology of osteoporosis and osteoporotic fractures. *Epidemiol Rev* 1985;7:178-208.

35. van den Kroonenberg A, Munih P, Weigent-Hayes M, et al: Hip impact pact velocities and body configurations for experimental falls from standing height. *Trans Orthop Res Soc* 1993;18:24.

36. Holliday PJ, Gryfe CI, Griggs GT, et al: Accidental falls of elderly people, in *Center for Studies in Aging Videotape*, 1989, University of Toronto.

37. Robinovitch SN, Hayes WC, McMahon TA: Prediction of femoral impact forces in falls on the hip. *J Biomech Eng* 1991;113:366-374.

38. Greenspan SL, Myers ER, Maitland LA, et al: Fall severity and bone mineral density predict hip fracture in the elderly. *JAMA* 1993, in press.

39. Wolf SL: Exploring novel interventions to reduce falls in older individuals, in Apple DF Jr, Hayes WC (eds): *Prevention of Falls and Hip Fractures in the Elderly*. Rosemont, IL, American Academy of Orthopaedic Surgeons, 1994, chap 12.

40. Lauritzen JB, Petersen MM, Lund B: Effect of external hip protectors on hip fractures. *Lancet* 1993;341:11-13.

41. Wallace RB, Ross JE, Huston JC, et al: Iowa FICSIT trial: The feasibility of elderly wearing a hip joint protective garment to reduce hip fractures. *J Am Geriatr Soc* 1993;41:338-340.

42. Sellberg MS, Huston JC, Kruger DH: The development of a passive protective device for the elderly to prevent hip fractures from accidental falls. *Adv Bioeng* 1992;22:505-508.

43. Huston JC, Sellberg MS, Kundel C, et al: A passive protective device to prevent hip fracture from falls in the elderly, in Apple DF Jr, Hayes WC (eds): *Prevention of Falls and Hip Fractures in the Elderly*. Rosemont, IL, American Academy of Orthopaedic Surgeons, 1994, chap 13.

44. Hayes WC, Robinovitch SN, McMahon TA: Energy-shunting hip padding system reduces femoral impact force from a simulated fall to below fracture threshold, in Yang K (ed): *Proceeding of the Third CDC Symposium on Injury Prevention Through Biomechanics*. Detroit, MI, Wayne State University, 1993, in press.

Chapter 6

Characteristics of Falls and Fallers and the Risk of Hip and Wrist Fracture

Michael C. Nevitt, PhD
Steven R. Cummings, MD

Hip fracture is the most medically devastating injury in older women, and associated health care costs are high. Wrist fractures are among the most common fracture types.[1] About 90% of hip fractures and wrist fractures occur as a result of falls.[2] Although much more potential energy may be available in a fall than is needed to fracture a hip or wrist in an older person,[3] only about 1% of falls cause hip fracture and about 5% result in any type of fracture.[4,5] In women, hip and wrist fractures have very different relationships to age: the incidence of hip fractures increases exponentially after about age 60, while the incidence of wrist fractures rises from age 50 to 65, then reaches a plateau after age 65.[6] This pattern suggests that there may be differences in the type of osteoporosis and the type and mechanisms of falls for these two fracture types. The rapid increase in the rate of hip fractures with age is not fully accounted for by increases in the number of falls or decreases in bone mass of the hip with age.[7,8] Therefore, other factors must increase the susceptibility to hip fractures.

When an older person falls, the nature of the fall and the characteristics of the faller may influence the risk and type of fracture. We have hypothesized[9] that the activity at the time of the fall, the direction and point of impact of the fall, factors that increase or attenuate the force of impact (such as protective responses and the energy-absorbing properties of impact surfaces), and the mineral density at the skeletal site of impact may all affect the risk that hip or wrist fracture will result from a fall.

In a previously published study,[10] these hypotheses were tested in case-control analyses nested in a large, prospective cohort study of community-dwelling older women. Women who fell and broke a hip or wrist were compared with a prospective sample of women who fell but did not sustain a fracture.

Table 1 Characteristics of falls and fallers associated with the risk of hip or wrist fracture

	Increased Risk	Decreased Risk
Hip fracture versus fall without fracture	Fall standing/turning/transfer Fall sideways/straight down Fall on hip/side of leg/buttocks Tallness Triceps weakness Fall on hard surface Decreased femoral neck bone density	Fall onto outstretched hand Grabbing or hitting objects during fall
Wrist fracture versus fall without fracture	Fall backward Fall onto outstretched hand Tallness Decreased distal radius bone density	Grabbing or hitting objects during fall

The main findings of these analyses are summarized in Table 1. The direction and point of impact of the fall were strongly associated with the risk of both hip and wrist fractures. Falls while standing or turning, falls sideways, straight down, with direct impact on the hip, side of the leg, or buttocks increased the risk of a hip fracture. Falls backward and falls onto a hand or wrist increased the risk of wrist fracture.

Factors that can increase or attenuate the fall's force of impact also affect the risk of hip or wrist fracture. In multivariate analyses comparing patients who fell on or near the hip but did not fracture it with those who fell and broke their hip, breaking the fall with an outstretched hand or grabbing or hitting an object on the way down decreased the risk of hip fracture, while tallness, falls onto a hard surface, and arm weakness were factors that increased risk of hip fracture. Among women who fell onto a hand or wrist, taller women had an increased risk of wrist fracture, while those who broke the momentum of the fall by grabbing or hitting an object had a decreased risk of wrist fracture. When a patient fell on or near the hip or landed on a hand or wrist, decreased bone mineral density at that site greatly increased the risk of fracture.

Among fallers who did not sustain a fracture, dangerous falls (falls sideways and falls onto or near the hip) were significantly more likely to occur while standing, turning, or descending stairs and were significantly less likely to occur while walking or running. Patients aged 75 and older were significantly less likely to use a hand to break a fall. No other falls characteristics differed by age.

Our findings suggest that the nature of the fall is important in determining the type of fracture that occurs, while factors that attenuate the force of impact of the fall and bone density determine whether a fracture will occur when a faller lands on a particular bone. Falling on or near the hip substantially increases the risk of hip fracture, while falling onto an outstretched hand decreases the risk of hip fracture and increases the risk of wrist fracture. Thus, age-related declines in strength and in the effectiveness of protective arm responses may account, in part, for the fact that the risk of hip fractures but not wrist fractures increases with patient age. Interventions designed to decrease the risk of falls through strength training and exercise programs may also be beneficial by improving protective responses during a fall, thus providing additional protection against the risk of hip fracture.

In this and another recent study,[11] falls sideways are associated with a greatly increased risk of hip fracture. Little is known about factors that influence the direction of a fall, but a better understanding of the determinants of fall direction may suggest new interventions to prevent hip fractures. Our findings also indicate that the risk of hip fractures, in particular, may be reduced by measures that attenuate the impact forces of a fall, such as the use of energy-absorbing flooring materials in places where elderly patients reside or the application of protective padding around the hip in women at risk for hip fracture.[11,12] Finally, preservation of bone mass in older women should reduce the risk of fracture in those prone to falling.

References

1. Cummings SR, Kelsey JL, Nevitt MC, et al: Epidemiology of osteoporosis and osteoporotic fractures. *Epidemiol Rev* 1985;7:178-208.
2. Melton LJ III, Chao EYS, Lane J: Biomechanical aspects of fractures, in Riggs BL, Melton LJ III (eds): *Osteoporosis: Etiology, Diagnosis, and Management*. New York, NY, Raven Press, 1988, pp 111-131.
3. Muckle DS, Bentley G, Deane G, et al: Basic sciences of the hip, in Muckle DS (ed): *Femoral Neck Fractures and Hip Joint Injuries*. New York, NY, John Wiley and Sons, 1977, pp 1-54.
4. Nevitt MC, Cummings SR, Kidd S, et al: Risk factors for recurrent nonsyncopal falls. *JAMA* 1989;261:2663-2668.
5. Tinetti ME, Speechley M, Gintner SF: Risk factors for falls among elderly persons living in the community. *N Engl J Med* 1988;319:1701-1707.
6. Melton LJ III: Epidemiology of fractures, in Riggs BL, Melton LJ III (eds): *Osteoporosis: Etiology, Diagnosis, and Management*. New York, NY, Raven Press, 1988, pp 133-154.
7. Horsman A, Burkinshaw L: Stochastic models of femoral bone loss and hip fracture risk, in Kleerekoper M, Krane SM (eds): *Clinical Disorders of Bone and Mineral Metabolism*. New York, NY, Mary Ann Liebert, Inc, 1989, pp 253-260.
8. Melton LJ III, Kan SH, Wahner HW, et al: Lifetime fracture risk: An approach to hip fracture risk assessment based on bone mineral density and age. *J Clin Epidemiol* 1988;41:985-994.
9. Cummings SR, Nevitt MC: A hypothesis: The causes of hip fractures. *J Gerontol* 1989;44:M107-111.
10. Nevitt MC, Cummings SR, Study of Osteoporotic Fractures Research Group: Type of fall and risk of hip and wrist fractures: The study of osteoporotic fractures. *J Am Geriatr Soc* 1993;41:1226-1234.
11. Lauritzen JB, Petersen MM, Lund B: Effect of external hip protectors on hip fractures. *Lancet* 1993;341:11-13.
12. Hayes WC, Myers ER, Morris JN, et al: Impact near the hip dominates fracture risk in elderly nursing home residents who fall. *Calcif Tissue Int* 1993;52:192-198.

Chapter 7

The Epidemiology of Falls and Hip Fractures Among Older Persons

Richard W. Sattin, MD, FACP

Falls and hip fractures among older persons rank as one of the most serious public health problems in the United States today, costing an estimated $10 billion per year in 1985.[1,2] The injury that can result from a fall can be considered a "disease" that has a short latency period and that results from the acute, rapid exposure to energy. The amount, distribution, duration, and rapidity of energy received and the person's response to the transfer of that energy can determine whether or not an injury will occur.[3] To estimate the magnitude of falls and hip fractures, data describing the epidemiology of fall deaths in the United States and nonfatal falls in general (and hip fractures in particular), along with potential areas for prevention, are presented here.

Fall-Related Mortality

The number of deaths from falls was determined by using data from annual mortality records compiled by the National Center for Health Statistics. Fall-related deaths were defined as those with an external underlying cause of death coded as E880-E888 according to the International Classification of Diseases, Ninth Revision. Rates were calculated using population estimates from the Bureau of the Census.

Falls are the leading cause of death resulting from injury among older persons, mainly because of the impact among those 85 years of age or older.[2] Among persons aged 65 to 84 years, falls are the second leading cause of death from injury for females and the third for males. More than half of injury-related deaths of women and one third of men aged 85 or older are a result of a fall (Fig. 1).

In 1989, there were 9,187 deaths from falls among persons aged 65 years or older. The rate of fall-related deaths rises markedly after age 75, for all races and both sexes. White men aged 85 years or older

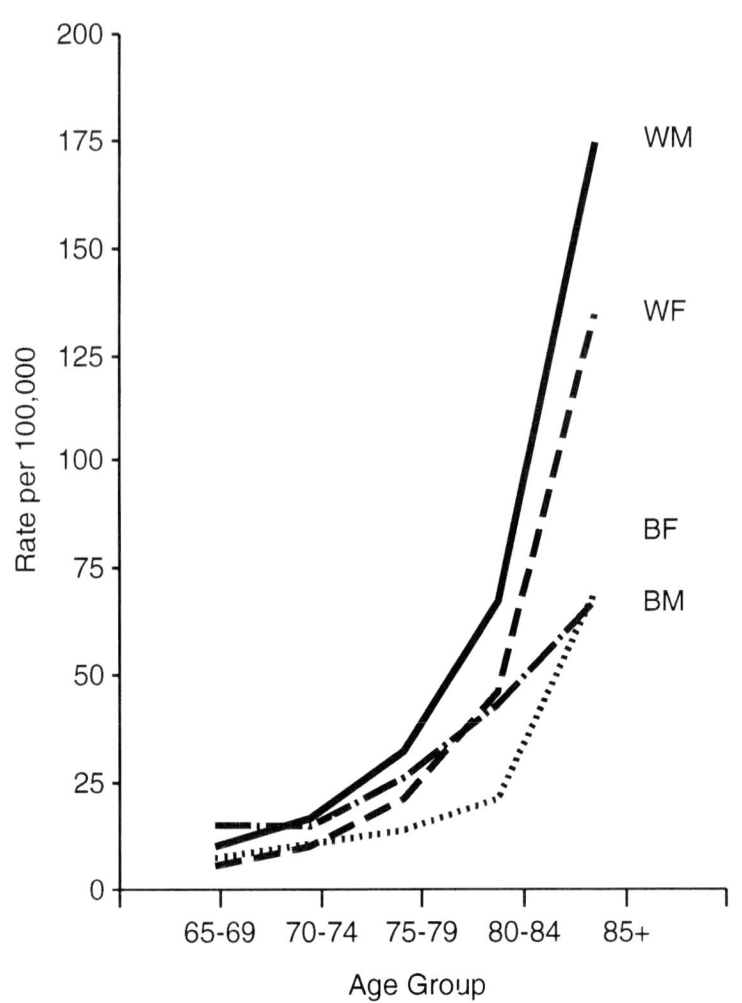

Fig. 1 *Fall death rates per 100,000 persons by age, sex, and race, United States, 1989.*

had the highest death rate, 176 per 100,000 persons in 1989. In fact, for persons aged 75 years or older, white men had the highest fall-related death rates.

The largest percentage of fall-related deaths among older persons occurred in the winter (26.9%); the fewest occurred in the summer (23.1%). However, the percentage of deaths by region did not vary considerably or consistently by season. Residents of the South actually had a higher proportion of deaths in winter than residents of other regions. This lack of consistency in seasonal occurrence is found in other years as well as in 1989.

Overall, about 45% of fall-related deaths among older persons occurred in the home and another 15% occurred in residential institutions. Even though the percentage of fall-related deaths occurring in the home declines with increasing age (above age 65, from 57% to 38%), there was a commensurate increase, from 7% to 19%, in the percentage of fall-related deaths occurring in nursing homes. Thus, the number of fall-related deaths occurring in places of residence remained fairly constant among older persons.

Mendlein and associates[4] compared data from 8,713 fall death cases with 1,438,872 controls where death was not injury-related to determine biologically plausible risk factors for fall mortality.[4] These factors might increase the risk of falling, severity of injury given that a fall had occurred, or risk of death after the fall. These data were adjusted for age, race, sex, autopsy status, hospitalization status, and number of medical conditions on death certificates. The medical conditions most prevalent per 100 fall deaths were pulmonary embolism (12.6), stroke (4.2), hypertension (3.3), diabetes (3.3), myocardial infarction (3.0), and anemia (1.3). Most striking is the prevalence odds ratio (POR) of 11.7 (95% confidence interval; 10.9 to 12.5) for pulmonary embolism, meaning that this condition was nearly 12 times more prevalent in fall death cases than in the controls.

At every age, the association between pulmonary embolism and fall deaths was about 1.5- to 2-fold greater for women than men. For both sexes, the POR increased with age (ages 65 to 74, POR 6.2 for men, and 11.0 for women; ages 75 to 84, POR 9.0 for men, and 13.8 for women; and ages 85 or older, POR 9.8 for men, and 18.5 for women).

Prevalence odds ratios ranged from 1.7 for deaths with no fractures to 19.1 for deaths with an upper limb fracture, 21.0 for deaths with a hip fracture, and 30.9 for deaths with a lower limb fracture other than hip. These data reiterate the need for clinical trials to determine the best type and most timely initiation of prophylactic therapies for deep venous thrombosis while balancing the risk of complications of bleeding associated with such therapy.

Fall-Related Morbidity

Figure 2 presents data from the National Health Interview Survey for all nonfatal injuries in the United States grouped by cause of injury.[5] In 1986, more than 11.5 million injuries were the result of falls. Motor vehicle traffic injuries were half as frequent as falls. Because of the survey design and the number of persons interviewed, these data could not be stratified by age, sex, or other important demographic variables.

The Centers for Disease Control and Prevention, together with the Florida Department of Health and Rehabilitative Services, conducted the population-based Study to Assess Falls Among the Elderly (SAFE) to determine the incidence of fall injury events among persons aged 65 years or older.[6,7] All hospitals serving this catchment area, the southern third of Miami Beach, Florida, were in-

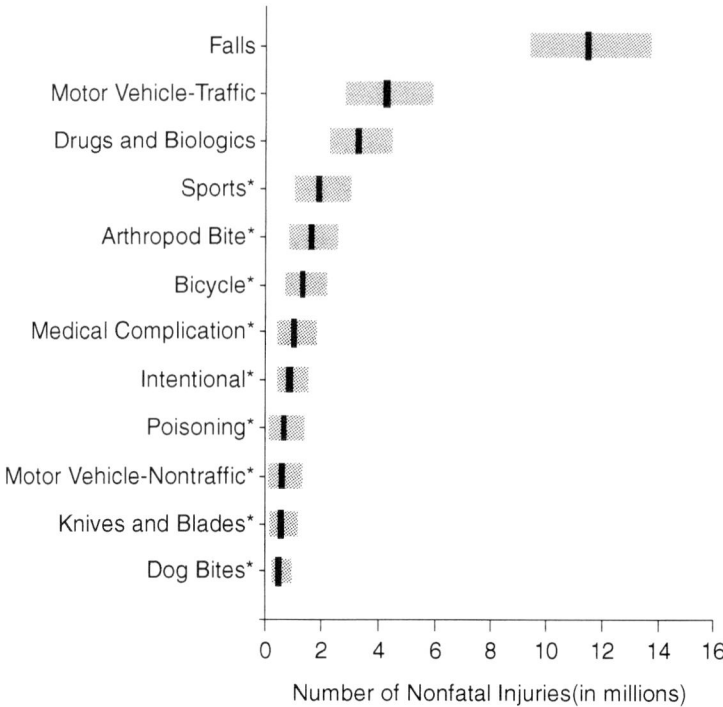

*Standard error > 20 percent of the estimate

Fig. 2 *Injuries for the civilian noninstitutionalized resident population by external causes, United States, 1986.*

cluded and the surveillance system included cause of injury codes. The data from SAFE are presented in Figure 3.

For men and women, the rate of falls and fall injuries increased exponentially by age. In men aged 65 to 69, this exponential increase reached a low of 25 per 1,000 persons; in women of the same age, the rate was 36 per 1,000 persons. In men and women aged 85 or older, the increase reached a high of 139 to 159, respectively, per 1,000 persons studied.

Compared with men, women tended to have higher rates per 1,000 persons per year of fractures of the upper limb (13.6 versus 4.4), hip (12.8 versus 6.0), neck or trunk (10.0 versus 5.3), and other lower limb (3.7 versus 1.6), but not of the skull (2.2 versus 2.2). Men tended to have the same or similar rate as women for open wounds to the head (15.1) and to the upper limb (2.4 versus 1.5), and for intracranial injuries (3.0 versus 3.1).

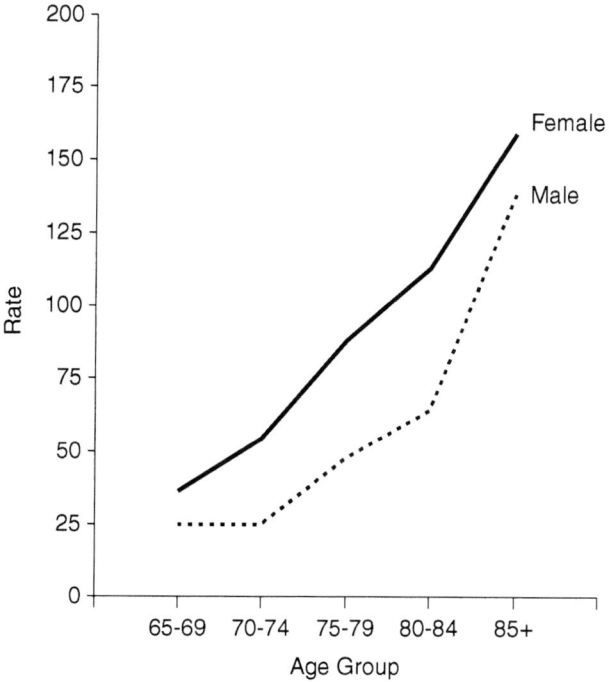

Fig. 3 *Age- and sex-specific rates of fall injury events by age and sex, Study to Assess Falls Among the Elderly (SAFE), Miami Beach, Florida, 1985-1987.*

All patients with a hip fracture were admitted to the hospital regardless of age. For persons with skull fracture/intracranial injury, or with other fractures or other injuries, the percentage of patients hospitalized increased fairly steadily by age. The variation in percentage of patients hospitalized reflects an increased prevalence of both cardiovascular and cerebrovascular ailments among persons who fell. The two most common concurrent medical diagnoses were syncope (15.6%) and conduction disorder/dysrhythmias (15.1%). Less frequently mentioned diagnoses included chronic ischemic heart disease (9.3%), anemia (8.7%), diabetes (8.3%), hypertensive disease (8.2%), acute/subacute ischemic heart disease (6.9%), and urinary tract infection (6.4%).

For those with hip fracture, conduction disorders (11.7%), chronic ischemic heart disease (11.4%), anemia (11.1%) and diabetes (7.8%) were the most common concurrent medical diagnoses, while syncope occurred much less frequently (2.5%).

The living arrangements of an older person hospitalized after a fall can be affected profoundly. Overall, 49% of all falls occurred within the home. About 62% of those persons who fell at home and were hospitalized for a hip fracture were discharged to a nursing home.

The data from the National Hospital Discharge Survey[8] can be used to estimate the incidence of hip fractures in the United States, even though the data for cause of injury are not available. The estimated number of hip fracture hospitalizations for persons aged 65 years or older for the years 1985 to 1990 are as follows: 1985, 238,000; 1986, 233,000; 1987, 233,000; 1988, 231,000; 1989, 243,000; and 1990, 261,000. Between 76% and 80% of these hip fractures occurred in women.

For all persons aged 65 years or older, the yearly rate of hip fracture hospitalizations has not noticeably changed between 1985 through 1990. For women, the rate remains between 100 and 120 per 10,000 persons, and for men, it remains about 40 per 10,000 persons (Fig. 4). Age- and sex-specific rates also show no noticeable change by year. Women aged 75 or older have the highest rates, around 200 per 10,000 persons, followed by men aged 75 years or older at around 100 per 10,000 persons (Fig. 5).

Obviously, current prevention strategies have not made an impact. One apparent bright spot has been the reduction of in-hospital hip fracture mortality (although this might partially reflect faster patient discharge). In 1970, the in-hospital mortality from hip fracture was 11.3%.[9] For the years 1985 through 1987, the in-hospital mortality rate had been reduced to 5.1% and for the years 1988 through 1990, it had been reduced further to 4.3%.[8]

These data from the National Hospital Discharge Survey, however, also suggest that undercounting of deaths caused by falls is a major problem. If the 4.3% of the 243,000 hip fractures occurred among persons aged 65 years or older in 1989, then 10,500 resulted in death during hospitalization. If 90% of these hip fracture-related deaths were caused by falls, it could be estimated that about 9,500 deaths caused by falls resulted from only one type of injury. Mortality data from 1989 reveal that 9,200 people aged 65 years or older died as a result of a fall-related injury.[8]

Risk Factors for Injurious Falls

Injuries can be viewed as a problem in medical ecology, that is, as a relationship between a person (the host), an agent, and the environment.[2,3]

Host Factors

Age and Sex With aging, physiologic changes occur in articular cartilage, bone, ligaments, and muscle.[10] During an injury event, these changes in the musculoskeletal system can lead to a decreased ability to withstand the effects of mechanical energy.

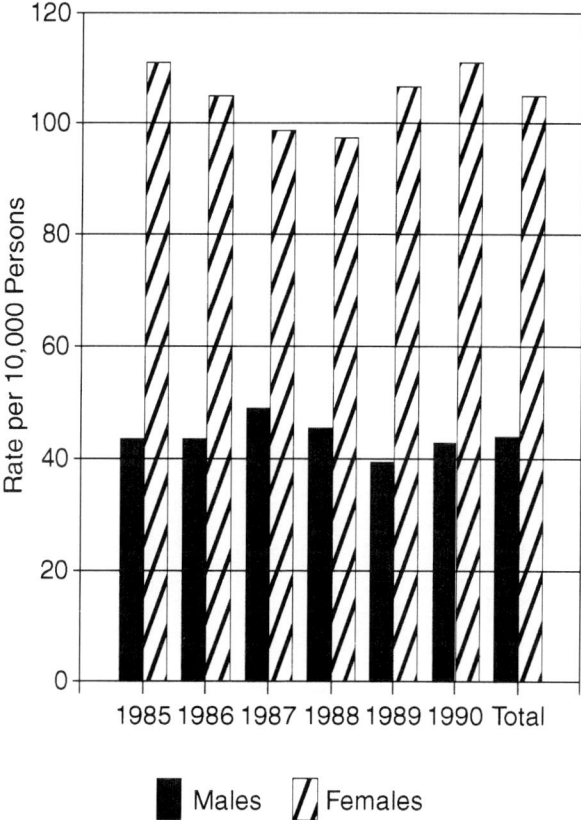

Fig. 4 *Rate of hip fracture hospitalization per 10,000 persons by sex and year, United States, 1985-1990.*

Women and men may have different outcomes from a fall for a number of reasons. For example, osteoporosis may play a substantial role in hip and other limb fractures for women.[11] On the other hand, women might fall differently than men and absorb mechanical energy at different parts of the body (for example, the hip in women, and the head in men).[7]

Chronic Diseases   Cerebrovascular, aardiovascular, and neurologic disorders are frequently associated with a fall.[12,13] Preventing and lessening the impact of these chronic ailments could lead to a substantial decrease in the future number of falls and fall-related injury among older persons.

Gait and Balance   Abnormal gait and balance have been repeatedly implicated as risk factors for falls among older persons.[13,14] Whether

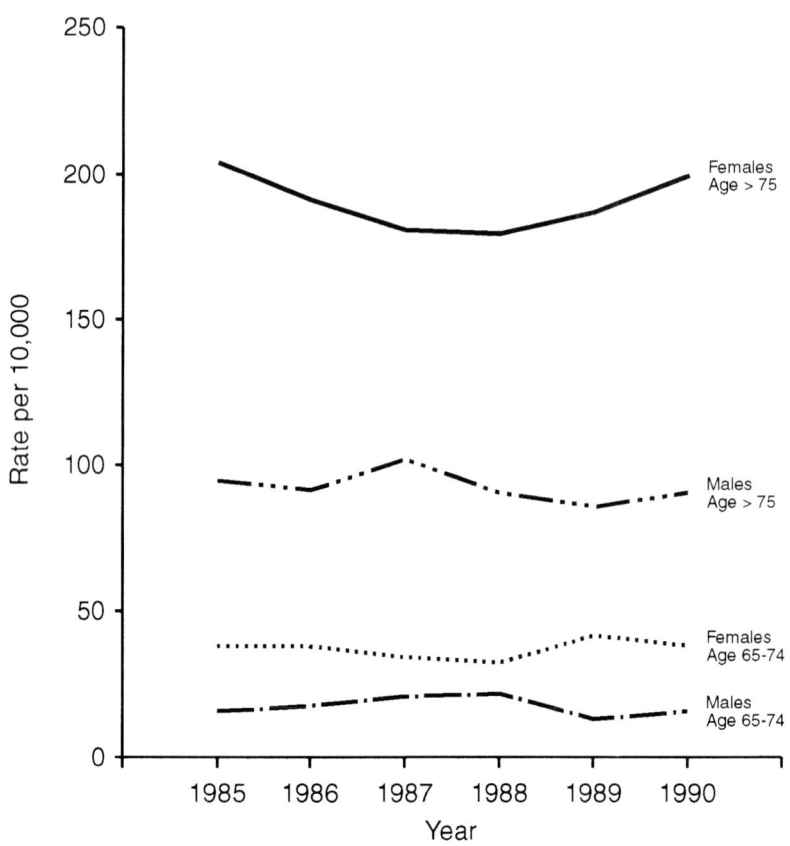

Fig. 5 *Rate of hip fracture hospitalization per 10,000 persons by age and sex, United States, 1985-1990.*

physical retraining through exercise, muscle strengthening, or some other mechanism will help to decrease fall injury events among the elderly is unknown.

Vision   Impaired visual acuity and depth perception have been associated with an increased risk of falls and hip fracture.[14,15] Early correction of these problems and detection and treatment of common conditions such as glaucoma and cataracts should improve visual function and might reduce falls.

Mental Status   Impaired mental status and depression are associated with an increased risk of falls and fall-related injury.[13,16] It is not known which interventions can reduce the incidence of fall-related injury and simultaneously maintain a high level of cognitive functioning in this high-risk patient group.

Medication Use   In the elderly person who takes psychotropic medication that has a long half-life, the risk of hip fracture is significantly increased.[17] Also, multiple drug use and its relation to fall incidence appears to be an important problem.[18] Effective reduction in physician prescribing practices for long half-life benzodiazepines is needed.

Alcohol Abuse   Alcohol abuse is frequently a factor in injury. Alcohol abuse has been associated frequently with falls in persons younger than 65 years of age, but most studies have not shown this association in elderly persons.[13,19] However, long-term abuse of alcohol can lead to various chronic medical conditions that increase risk of falls or fall-related injury.

Agent Factors

Very little is known about the mechanism or transfer of energy during a fall.[3] Mechanical energy is the most common agent of injury related to falls among older people. By better understanding these responses to impact, protective devices, such as hip pads, can be developed for high-risk persons. These devices could lead to the energy load being transmitted at a slower velocity or dissipated over a much larger area, thus preventing an injury if a fall occurred.

Environmental Factors

The environment has been implicated in one third to one half of all falls or fall-related injuries.[20,21] Recommended solutions have included improvements in lighting; redesign of stairs; removal of throw rugs; use of slip-resistant stripping in bathtubs; proper placement of shelving; improvements in shoe design; and improved streets and walkways. These recommendations make intuitive sense, but nearly all of the studies on which these recommendations are based have not determined if those "hazards" are as prevalent in the homes of persons who did not fall as in the homes of those who did. Although environmental hazards probably contribute to falls and fall-related injury in the elderly, the extent of this contribution, how multiple potential hazards interact, and how this effect is modified by host and agent factors is unknown.

Prevention

Although much has been learned over the last decade about the causes of falls, still little is known about the most effective ways of preventing them. Fall prevention efforts need to be directed not only toward older persons but younger persons as well. Injury control prevention strategies can be conceptualized by separating the injury event into three distinct phases: preevent, event, and postevent.[22]

Outline 1 Possible elements of a public health program to prevent falls among the elderly

Preevent
    Exercise promotion and physical conditioning
    Cessation of smoking and excessive use of alcohol
    Nutrition education
    Reduction of psychotropic medication use
    Regular eye examinations
    Osteoporosis prevention
    Hazard evaluation and modification of residential institutions
    Home hazard awareness
    Use of proper footwear
    Safe outdoor walk routes during all weather conditions

Event
    Energy-absorbing flooring for high-risk areas
    Hip protection devices for high-risk persons

Postevent
    Emergency response call systems or buddy systems
    Improvements in emergency communication systems
    Health promotion and hazard prevention (all elements listed under Preevent)

For example, the preevent phase of injury might be affected by targeting young people with programs that promote smoking cessation, exercise, and reduction in alcohol use. These programs would lead to a reduction in chronic diseases and their potential outcomes—falls. Teaching both middle-aged men and women about the need to maintain physical fitness and bone strength may reduce future injuries. If exercise and general muscle conditioning for the elderly prove effective, health practitioners could include these programs as well. Teaching both perimenopausal and older women about general nutrition, calcium intake, and the potential benefits and risks associated with estrogen use may reduce future injuries. For older persons, the number of hip fractures and other fall-related injuries may be reduced by altering medication use, providing regular eye examinations and treatment for eye disorders, making homes and residential institutions safer, altering shoe design, and maintaining safe outdoor walk routes during all weather conditions (Outline 1).

Technologic development of energy-absorbing flooring and the development of easily worn, unobtrusive hip protection would be useful in managing the event phase of injury. For the postevent stage, a network of emergency response call buttons or buddy systems could improve overall survival in older persons who do fall but cannot get help quickly. Improved care for older persons who have been injured, including improved methods of prophylaxis from deep venous thrombosis, might reduce the overall disability and incidence of mortality. Finally, it is important to continue health promotion and hazard prevention after a person has fallen.

In conclusion, empirically-derived interventions must be used until effective prevention modalities are developed for older persons. Clearly, more work is needed to improve the acute care treatment, management, and rehabilitation of patients injured in falls and to determine which interventions can decrease the risk of a fall or fall-related injury.

References

1. Rice DP, Mackenzie EJ, et al: *Cost of Injury in the United States: A Report to Congress, 1989*. San Francisco, CA, Institute for Health and Aging, University of California, 1989.

2. Sattin RW: Falls among older persons: A public health perspective. *Ann Rev Pub Health* 1992;13:489-508.

3. Committee on Trauma Research, Commission on Life Sciences, National Research Council, and the Institute of Medicine: *Injury in America: A Continuing Public Health Problem*. Washington, DC, National Academy Press, 1985, pp 25-36, 38-64.

4. Mendlein JM, Sattin RW, Waxweiler RJ, et al: Fall mortality and related medical conditions in the elderly: The association with pulmonary embolism. *J Aging Health* 1990;2:326-340.

5. Sosin DM, Sacks JJ, Sattin RW: Causes of nonfatal injuries in the United States, 1986. *Accid Anal Prev* 1992;24:685-687.

6. DeVito CA, Lambert DA, Sattin RW, et al: Fall injuries among the elderly: Community-based surveillance. *J Am Geriatr Soc* 1988;36:1029-1035.

7. Sattin RW, Lambert-Huber DA, DeVito CA, et al: The incidence of fall injury events among the elderly in a defined population. *Am J Epidemiol* 1990;131:1028-1037.

8. National Center for Health Statistics, 1985 to 1990.

9. Rodriguez JG, Sattin RW, Waxweiler RJ: Incidence of hip fractures, United States, 1970-1983. *Am J Prev Med* 1989;5:175-181.

10. States JD: Musculo-skeletal system impairment related to safety and comfort of drivers 55+, in Malfetti JL (ed): *Drivers 55+: Needs and Problems of Older Drivers: Survey Results and Recommendations, Proceedings of the Older Driver Colloquium, Orlando, Feb 4-7, 1985*. Falls Church, VA, AAA Foundation for Traffic Safety, 1985, pp 63-76.

11. Cummings SR, Kelsey JL, Nevitt MC, et al: Epidemiology of osteoporosis and osteoporotic fractures. *Epidemiol Rev* 1985;7:178-208.

12. Tinetti ME, Speechley M: Prevention of falls among the elderly. *N Engl J Med* 1989;320:1055-1059.

13. Tinetti ME, Speechley M, Ginter SF: Risk factors for falls among elderly persons living in the community. *N Engl J Med* 1988:319:1701-1707.

14. Nevitt MC, Cummings SR, Kidd S, et al: Risk factors for recurrent nonsyncopal falls: A prospective study. *JAMA* 1989;261:2663-2668.

15. Felson DT, Anderson JJ, Hannan MT, et al: Impaired vision and hip fracture: The Framingham Study. *J Am Geriatr Soc* 1989;37:495-500.

16. Campbell AJ, Reinken J, Allan BC, et al: Falls in old age: A study of frequencies and related clinical factors. *Age Ageing* 1981;10:264-270.

17. Ray WA, Griffin MR, Schaffner W, et al: Psychotropic drug use and the risk of hip fracture. *N Engl J Med* 1987;316:363-369.

18. Buchner DM, Larson EB: Falls and fractures in patients with Alzheimer-type dementia. *JAMA* 1987;257:1492-1495.

19. Nelson DE, Sattin RW, Langlois JA, et al: Alcohol as a risk factor for fall injury events among elderly persons living in the community. *J Am Geriatr Soc* 1992;40:658-661.

20. Lucht U: A prospective study of accidental falls and resulting injuries in the home among elderly people. *Acta Socio-Med Scand* 1971;3:105-120.
21. Rubenstein LZ, Robbins AS, Schulman BL, et al: Falls and instability in the elderly. *J Am Geriatr Soc* 1988;36:266-278.
22. Haddon W Jr, Baker SP: Injury control, in Clark DW, MacMahion B (eds): *Preventive and Community Medicine*, ed 2. Boston, MA, Little Brown and Co, 1981, pp 109-140.

Section Three

Treatment

Chapter 8

Functional Outcome of Hip Fractures in the Elderly

James E. Carpenter, MD
Elizabeth R. Myers, PhD
Tobin N. Gerhart, MD
Harris S. Yett, MD
John N. Morris, PhD
Wilson C. Hayes, PhD

Introduction

Hip fractures, which occur primarily in the elderly, have enormous social and economic impact. The incidence of hip fracture in the United States has been estimated at 250,000 cases per year. As the population ages, this incidence may rise to as high as 500,000 cases per year by the end of the century.[1] Annual costs attributable to this injury are estimated to be over $7 billion.[1-6] Despite these high frequencies and costs, there is no well-accepted method for evaluating treatment outcome. Traditionally, treatment has been evaluated on the basis of mortality,[7,8] complications of treatment,[9] or radiographic findings.[10-13] The reporting of functional results could provide a better understanding of the impact of hip fractures and treatment effectiveness. Previously, functional evaluation of patients with hip fractures has generally been limited to gross measures of ambulatory status.[14-16] Other evaluation instruments, based on activities of daily living (ADL), have been designed for patients with chronic disease.[17,18] Therefore, a system that isolates hip-related function when evaluating the outcome of hip fracture treatment is preferred.

Since the introduction of hip arthroplasty, many objective rating systems have been proposed for evaluation of reconstructive surgery of the hip.[19-24] Some of these have been extended to evaluate hip fracture outcome as well.[25-27] Because the hip fracture patient population differs from the arthroplasty population, the instruments used to assess hip arthroplasty outcome are not well suited for evaluating hip fracture outcome. In an effort to improve outcome reporting in hip fracture patients, we developed a new scoring instrument, specifically for hip fracture patients, that was intended to evaluate the impact of hip fracture on subsequent patient function. It was designed so that it can be used to determine baseline functional abilities in patients with acute hip fractures, and, at the same time, allow follow-up based on data collected over the telephone. In contrast to the arthroplasty rating scales, there is no scoring of hip motion or deformity, hip pain accounts for a small (15%) portion of the total score, ambulation and ADL account for over two thirds of the score (70%), and a mental status evaluation (10%) is included.

Methods

The hip fracture evaluation instrument is a simple scoring system of up to 100 points (Table 1). It does not require patient examination, functional testing, or radiographs. Fifty points are allotted for evaluation of ambulation; these include up to 20 points used for walking on level ground, up to 15 points for stair climbing and more vigorous activity, up to 10 points for not using walking aids, and up to 5 points for absence of limping. Of the remaining 50 points, 20 are used for evaluation of ADL (feeding, bathing, dressing, bowel and bladder function). Up to 4 points are allowed for each of these activities. Fifteen points are allotted for hip pain evaluation, 5 points for lack of decubitus skin breakdown, and 10 points for assessment of mental status. Points for each of these sections are given on a continuous scale, rather than all or none; thus, any score from 0 to 100 is possible.

The instrument was validated in a randomly selected cohort of 421 residents from the Hebrew Rehabilitation Center for Aged (HRCA) in Boston. The HRCA is an extended-care facility providing nursing and other clinical services for a wide range of care levels. Data were collected sufficient for evaluation of each patient according to our new scoring instrument and five other instruments that were believed to be representative of the broad spectrum of ADL-based indices used to characterize the functional status of elderly patients in nursing facilities. Statistical analysis of the data was performed with correlational comparisons of the five scales to the new scoring instrument.

The instrument was also used to study 210 patients with acute femoral neck fractures at Beth Israel Hospital in Boston from Jan 1, 1985 to Dec 31, 1987.[28] During their hospitalization (usually after their surgery), an assessment of preinjury functional status was obtained for all patients by a trained physical therapist. Follow-up assessments of functional status and medical condition were performed using the same hip fracture scoring instrument and a questionnaire by telephone interview with the patient, a family member, or caretaker (including nursing home staff) after a minimum of one year. Each patient's hospital medical record was reviewed retrospectively for preoperative risk factors that might pre-

Table 1 Functional status instrument designed for evaluation of elderly patients with hip fractures

Hip Fracture Evaluation Score

		Points
Ambulation		0-50
Level ground	0 to 20 points	
Bedridden	0 pt	
Bed to chair	5 pt	
Walks with 2 assists	10 pt	
Walks with 1 assist	15 pt	
Walks independently	20 pt	
Activity level	0 to 15 points	
Unable to climb stairs	0 pt	
Able to climb stairs	5 pt	
Walks 5 blocks	10 pt	
and climbs stairs	10 pt	
Vigorous activity	15 pt	
Walking aids	0 to 10 points	
Walker/2 crutches	0 pt	
Cane	5 pt	
Walks with no aids	10 pt	
Limp	0 to 5 points	
Limps	0 pt	
No limp	5 pt	
Activities of Daily Living		0-20
Feeding	4 pt	
Bathing	4 pt	
Dressing	4 pt	
Bladder care	4 pt	
Bowel care	4 pt	
Hip Pain		0-15
Constant	0 pt	
Takes pain medication	5 pt	
Complains of pain	10 pt	
No pain	15 pt	
Mental Status		0-10
Persistently disoriented	0 pt	
No confusion	10 pt	
Skin		0-5
Decubitus breakdown	0 pt	
No decubitus breakdown	5 pt	
		100 Points

dict poor outcome and for in-hospital complications of treatment. The risk factors studied were age, cerebral dysfunction, and comorbidities.

Of the 209 patients with femoral neck fractures treated surgically (1 patient was treated nonsurgically), 21 were under the age of 60 years and were excluded from follow-up, 36 died within the first year following the fracture, 11 died after one year but before follow-up assessments could be made, 2 had errors in their preinjury evaluations and were excluded from follow-up, and 1 patient was lost and no follow-up data were available. The remaining 138 patients, the outcome study group, had follow-up assessments one year or more after their fractures with a range of one to five years and a mean of 2.8 years.

The functional status score at the time of follow-up was analyzed according to its dependence on preoperative factors (age, comorbidities, cerebral dysfunction, preinjury functional status) and type of surgery. Of the 138 patients, 29 were treated with internal fixation, 37 with an uncemented Austin-Moore prosthesis, and 72 with a cemented bipolar prosthesis. There was no difference in fracture patterns between the patients treated with a Moore prosthesis and those treated with a bipolar prosthesis.

Results

The correlations between our assessment instrument and the five ADL-based indices evaluated in the 421 HRCA residents ranged from a low of 0.68 for the Uniscale Quality of Life Index to a high of 0.88 for the Katz Activities of Daily Living scale and for the ADL Component of RUGII. Evaluation of the components of the total score showed highest correlations for ADL (0.48 to 0.94), ambulatory function (0.61 to 0.83), and mental status (0.06 to 0.68). Presence or absence of pressure sores (0.17 to 0.25) and pain (0.01 to 0.06) in the hip did not correlate well with the functional status indicators, while evaluation of use of equipment was intermediate in its correlation (0.30 to 0.53). These results suggest that the new hip fracture scoring instrument can reliably measure functional status in elderly patients according to these previously published functional status indicators.

Average follow-up was 2.8 years (range: 1.1 to 5.0 years). The in-hospital length of stay varied widely, from a minimum of 4 days to a maximum of 179 days. By one-way analysis of variance (ANOVA), the average length of stay for each treatment group was not significantly different, with 17.8 days in the internal fixation group, 17.7 days in the Moore group, and 15.8 days in the bipolar group. The mean number of in-hospital complications for each group was 0.38 in the internal fixation group, 0.62 in the Moore group, and 0.51 in the bipolar group. These did not differ statistically by one-way ANOVA. The percentage of patients requiring some sort of reoperation for their hip fracture was 28% for the internal fixation group, 5% for the Moore group, and 3% for the bipolar group. The difference between the internal fixation and prosthesis groups was statistically significant ($p < 0.0005$). The reasons for reoperation in these patients are listed in Table 2.

The follow-up functional status ranged from a low of 20 to a high of 100 on the same 100-point assessment scale used for analysis of preoperative function. The internal fixation group had the highest follow-up score at 72.7, the bipolar group was intermediate at 69.1, and the Moore group had the lowest follow-up score at 57.3. By anal-

Table 2 Reoperations following initial treatment of 138 patients with femoral neck fractures

Treatment Group	Reason for Reoperation	Type of Reoperation
Internal fixation	Painful hardware	Pins removed
	Painful hardware	Pins removed
	Painful hardware	Pins removed
	Loss of reduction	Revision to bipolar
	Loss of reduction	Revision to bipolar
	Loss of reduction	Revision to bipolar
	Loss of reduction	Revision to THA*
	Loss of reduction	Revision to THA
	Osteonecrosis, collapse	Revision to THA
Moore prosthesis	Fracture below prosthesis	Long stem revision bipolar
Cemented	Infection	Girdlestone
bipolar	Dislocation	Open reduction
prosthesis		

*THA, total hip arthroplasty.

ysis of covariance (ANCOVA), the follow-up functional status depended strongly on preinjury functional status (p <0.0005). Age at the time of fracture and presence and absence of dementia were also significantly associated with functional status at follow-up (p <0.001 and p <0.05, respectively). Despite the differences between the follow-up functional scores in the treatment groups, when analyzed in light of their preexisting condition, the type of treatment had no significant effect on the functional score at the time of follow-up (p = 0.52).

Discussion

These data demonstrate the importance of the preoperative risk factors when studying outcome in hip fracture populations. If baseline functional status is not taken into account, it could be concluded that the type of surgical treatment makes a significant difference in outcome. However, when baseline functional status is included in analysis, age, preinjury functional status, and cerebral function are the only statistically significant factors in predicting functional outcome following femoral neck fractures. At a mean of 2.8 years follow-up, there was no basis for performing cemented, bipolar hemiarthroplasty versus uncemented Austin-Moore hemiarthroplasties. This has significant implications for reducing cost of hip fracture treatment, because the Austin-Moore prostheses are less costly than cemented bipolar prostheses.

In summary, this new method for evaluation of hip fracture outcome is based on a functional analysis instrument that can be used in elderly patients to obtain a prefracture assessment. Follow-up assessments can be made by telephone and evaluated with reference to the prefracture status. The assessment scale is correlated well with several ADL-based indices. When used to evaluate functional outcome in 138 patients with femoral neck fractures, age, mental status, and prefracture functional status were found to be important determinants of outcome, whereas the type of surgical treatment was not.

Acknowledgments

This work was supported by CDC grant CC102550 and by the Maurice E. Mueller Professorship in Biomechanics at Harvard Medical School (WCH).

References

1. Lindsay R, Dempster DW, Clemens T, et al: Incidence, cost, and risk factors of fracture of the proximal femur in the U.S.A., in Christiansen C, Arnaud CD, Nordin BEC, et al (eds): *Osteoporosis: Proceedings of the Copenhagen International Symposium on Osteoporosis*. Copenhagen, Denmark, Glostrup Hospital, Department of Clinical Chemistry, 1984, vol 1.

2. Kelsey JL: The epidemiology of diseases of the hip: A review of the literature. *Int J Epidemiol* 1977;6:269-280.

3. Riggs BL, Melton LJ III: Involutional osteoporosis. *N Engl J Med* 1986;314:1676-1686.

4. Jensen JS, Tøndevold E, Sørensen PH: Social rehabilitation following hip fractures. *Acta Orthop Scand* 1979;50:777-785.

5. Thomas TG, Stevens RS: Social effects of fractures of the neck of the femur. *Br Med J* 1974;3:456-458.

6. Ceder L, Ekelund L, Inerot S, et al: Rehabilitation after hip fracture in the elderly. *Acta Orthop Scand* 1979;50:681-688.

7. Miller CW: Survival and ambulation following hip fracture. *J Bone Joint Surg* 1978;60A:930-934.

8. Fitts WT Jr, Lehr HB, Schor S, et al: Life expectancy after fracture of the hip. *Surg Gynecol Obstet* 1959;108:7-12.

9. Johnson JTH, Crothers O: Nailing versus prosthesis for femoral-neck fractures: A critical review of long-term results in 239 consecutive private patients. *J Bone Joint Surg* 1975;57A:686-692.

10. Garden RS: Low-angle fixation in fractures of the femoral neck. *J Bone Joint Surg* 1961;43B:647-663.

11. Hunter GA: Should we abandon primary prosthetic replacement for fresh displaced fractures of the neck of the femur? *Clin Orthop* 1980;152:158-161.

12. Holmberg H, Kaln R, Thorngren K-G: Treatment and outcome of femoral neck fractures: An analysis of 2,418 patients admitted from their own homes. *Clin Orthop* 1987;218:42-52.

13. Barnes R, Brown JT, Garden RS, et al: Subcapital fractures of the femur: A prospective review. *J Bone Joint Surg* 1976;58B:2-24.

14. Gossling HR, Hardy JH: Fracture of the femoral neck: A comparative study of methods of treatment in 400 consecutive cases. *J Trauma* 1969;9:423-429.

15. Niemann KM, Mankin HJ: Fractures about the hip in an institutionalized patient population: II. Survival and ability to walk again. *J Bone Joint Surg* 1968;50A:1327-1340.

16. Sikorski JM, Barrington R: Internal fixation versus hemiarthroplasty for the displaced subcapital fracture of the femur: A prospective randomised study. *J Bone Joint Surg* 1981;63B:357-361.

17. Jette AM, Harris BA, Cleary PD, et al: Functional recovery after hip fracture. *Arch Phys Med Rehabil* 1987;68:735-740.

18. Mossey JM, Mutran E, Knott K, et al: Determinants of recovery 12 months after hip fracture: The importance of psychosocial factors. *Am J Public Health* 1989;79:279-286.

19. Judet R, Judet J: Technique and results with the acrylic femoral head prosthesis. *J Bone Joint Surg* 1952;34B:173-180.

20. D'Aubigné RM, Postel M: Functional results of hip arthroplasty with acrylic prosthesis. *J Bone Joint Surg* 1954;36A:451-475.

21. Shepherd MM: Assessment of function after arthroplasty of the hip. *J Bone Joint Surg* 1954;36B:354-363.

22. Charnley J: The long-term results of low-friction arthroplasty of the hip performed as a primary intervention. *J Bone Joint Surg* 1972;54B:61-76.

23. Harris WH: Traumatic arthritis of the hip after dislocation and acetabular fractures: Treatment by mold arthroplasty: An end-result study using a new method of result evaluation. *J Bone Joint Surg* 1969;51A:737-755.

24. Larson CB: Rating scale for hip disabilities. *Clin Orthop* 1963;31:85-93.

25. Greenough CG, Jones JR: Primary total hip replacement for displaced subcapital fracture of the femur. *J Bone Joint Surg* 1988;70B:639-643.

26. Salvati EA, Wilson PD Jr: Long-term results of femoral-head replacement. *J Bone Joint Surg* 1973;55A:516-524.

27. Lausten GS, Vedel P, Nielsen P-M: Fractures of the femoral neck treated with a bipolar endoprosthesis. *Clin Orthop* 1987;218:63-67.

28. Carpenter JE, Myers ER, Gerhart TN, et al: Functional outcome following femoral neck fractures in the elderly. *Orthop Trans* 1992;16:750.

Chapter 9

Treatment of Extracapsular Hip Fractures

Peter G. Trafton, MD

Significance of Extracapsular Hip Fractures

Because of differences in prognosis and treatment, hip fractures are separated into two basic categories: intracapsular and extracapsular. Intracapsular fractures, which will not be discussed in depth here, involve the anatomic femoral neck. The capsule of the hip joint attaches to the base of the neck, the broader metaphyseal region, including the lateral greater trochanter where the hip abductor muscles attach, and the medial lesser trochanter, the insertion of the iliopsoas (flexors). Extracapsular fractures occur in this region, generally, outside of the joint capsule. They represent approximately half of all "hip" fractures. Most extracapsular fractures are the result of low-energy trauma in elderly patients with osteoporosis. Substantially greater force is required to produce a similar injury in normal bone. Somewhat different concerns and treatment protocols are required for extracapsular fractures caused by high-energy trauma.

There are two major types of extracapsular fractures: intertrochanteric and subtrochanteric. Criteria to distinguish one from the other are neither well-delineated nor consistently applied. The distinction is less important now that current fixation techniques are reliable for the majority of extracapsular fractures.

The socioeconomic consequences of extracapsular hip fractures in the elderly parallel those of the intracapsular variety, with costly care, functional impairment, and well-recognized morbidity and mortality.[1] Increasing numbers of hip fractures, related to the absolute increase in the elderly population, and possibly to increasing incidence rates as well, underscore the seriousness of "hip fracture disease," and the benefits obtainable from its prevention. While treatment of the fracture and its associated medical problems is not fail-safe, this review seeks to emphasize that opportunities for significant improvements in outcome or cost reduction are unlikely to approach the yield of effective preventive measures.

Goals of Treatment for Hip Fractures

Nearly 45 years ago, Evans[2] pointed out that the primary goal of treatment was "preserving the life and general health in aged people whose fracture was but an incident in their general decline, while combining humane and efficient care with conservation of (available resources)." Therefore, treatment should relieve pain, avoid medical and surgical complications, and restore as much mobility as possible. Surgery is almost always the best way to achieve an optimal outcome, but it is only a part of the story.

Systems for Comprehensive, Multidisciplinary Care of Hip Fractures in the Elderly

It has been clearly demonstrated by Zuckerman[3,4] and others that an organized, systematic approach is a very successful way of providing comprehensive, multidisciplinary evaluation and care for elderly patients with hip fractures. While surgery may be the most obvious aspect of acute care for the patient with hip fracture, failure to recognize and effectively address the important additional issues may increase complications and compromise outcome. Furthermore, clarification of all the involved issues allows early goal-setting, which aids in the formulation of a patient's individualized treatment plan, and helps avoid inappropriate efforts to achieve unattainable walking ability or living arrangements. Issues that must be addressed include the patient's cognitive and emotional status, vision and hearing, cardiorespiratory function, nutrition and gastrointestinal function, endocrine disorders, urinary functions, other musculoskeletal problems, and baseline strength and endurance, as well as possible acute or chronic alterations in skin integrity and coagulopathy. The patient's social and family setting may provide crucial opportunities or limitations for rehabilitation after hip fracture. Optimal efficiency is provided by a multidisciplinary team for both evaluation and treatment. The composition of the team will depend on institutional and community resources.

Problems of Extracapsular Fractures

The trochanteric region connects the medially located femoral head with the more lateral shaft. Mechanical analyses and force-recording prostheses have shown that this region must withstand a threefold to fourfold increase in the body's weight during many activities, including attempts to lift the leg from a bed surface, or to get on and off a bedpan. A successful repair of a trochanteric fracture must resist such forces and maintain fracture alignment until union is achieved. Although precise restoration of anatomy is not essential, the overall configuration of the region is important for normal gait, as the local anatomy affects muscle function and leg length. Because of a well-vascularized, cancellous bone composition, fractures in this region almost always heal. However, without internal fixation, three to four months are typically required before the healing fracture callus is stable enough to avoid plastic deformation. Osteoporosis, along with falls, contributes to the risk of hip fracture. More importantly, it poses significant problems to the surgeon, because bone of poor mechanical quality is more prone to fixation failure.

Classification of Extracapsular Fractures

No clear boundary separates intertrochanteric from subtrochanteric fractures. A spectrum of injuries involves this area. A given fracture may be called intertrochanteric by one surgeon, and subtrochanteric by another. The distal limit of subtrochanteric fractures has also been variously defined. It is perhaps helpful to recall that classification systems were typically developed to predict the response of fractures to fixation with a given type of implant. Thus, Fielding's classification of subtrochanteric fractures according to location distal to the lesser trochanter predicted the risk of failure after fixation with a Jewett nail. Newer styles of fixation may render such a classification obsolete. Fixation failure was a significant concern in unstable intertrochanteric fractures (those with a large posteromedial comminuted fragment) until sliding hip screws replaced one-piece implants such as Jewett nails. Two-part sliding screws are not only stronger, but also permit the proximal and distal fracture fragments to settle into more stable contact with one another, so that the bone bears more of the load across the healing fracture site. Fixation failure is now much less frequent, and special reduction techniques such as medial displacement osteotomy are no longer needed.

Intertrochanteric fractures involve primarily the region bounded by the greater and lesser trochanters. Classification schemes for intertrochanteric fractures generally seek to predict instability, that is, the risk of displacement after fixation.[5] This increases with comminution, especially when a large displaced fragment involves the posteromedial area of the lesser trochanter. Displacement involving both trochanters (four-part fractures) results in more instability than when only one is involved (three-part fractures). So-called basilar neck fractures occur at the capsular attachment, where the femoral neck flares to join the trochanters. They are relatively infrequent, and are similar to other intertrochanteric fractures in problems and treatment.

Treatment of Extracapsular Fractures: The Patient

Management of hip fractures can be divided into treatment for the patient and for the fracture itself. Treatment of the patient, which is truly more important, begins with a thorough preoperative assessment and institution of a comprehensive, ongoing plan for management of all problems. Several issues deserve special emphasis. Nutritional deficits are so common in the elderly that routine diet supplements have been shown to reduce the risk of medical and wound-healing complications, and to expedite recovery. The risk of wound infection during surgery is further reduced by a short course of perioperative antibiotics, typically a first-generation cephalosporin begun with anesthesia induction and continued no longer than 24 to 48 hours. Deep venous thrombosis and pulmonary embolism are also significant risks for elderly patients with hip fractures, and various prophylactic regimens have been shown to produce a cost-effective reduction of risk. Geriatric psychiatric screening and care can reduce the chances that depression will limit the patient's potential for recovery.[6]

Physical rehabilitation is essential, focusing on moving the patient out of bed safely, with early transfer and gait training (usually with a walker for support). This assistance helps avoid excessive stress on the repaired fracture, and helps prevent falls, which can cause additional injuries. The patient's ability to perform necessary activities of daily living must be assessed, and provisions made for assistance with any needs that the patient cannot meet independently. Comparing such needs with the patient's capabilities results in effective discharge planning. This is most efficient when begun soon after hospitalization, based on expected goals that can be predicted from the patient's status prior to fracture. It is important to continue active rehabilitation efforts long enough to ensure attainment of realistic goals and maintenance of the patient's capabilities. At least six months are required before recovery from a hip fracture reaches a plateau.[7]

Treatment of Extracapsular Fractures: The Fracture

Focusing now on the fracture, it should be noted that extracapsular fractures, unlike the intracapsular variety, almost always unite, and osteonecrosis is rare. Surgical fracture fixation is done to maintain alignment while permitting mobilization of the patient. It is now the treatment of choice for almost all previously ambulatory patients with extracapsular hip fractures.

Nonsurgical treatment may be considered in two separate situations. The first is in the patient with no need for fracture reduction. The risk of systemic surgical complications is high in frail, nonambulatory patients with marked osteoporosis. Because walking is not an issue for these patients, hip deformity is acceptable. Fixation failure is likely, because of the extreme osteoporosis. Within a few days, such patients' fractures become less painful, and they can be managed comfortably with usual nursing measures for bedridden patients. The fracture is effectively ignored, except for initial analgesia and increased attention to prevention of pressure sores.

The second scenario for nonsurgical management is the ambulatory patient for whom fracture reduction is functionally important. Skeletal traction reliably provides and maintains an acceptable reduction for most extracapsular fractures, but must be continued for three or four months to avoid late loss of alignment. For many years, this was the standard treatment for extracapsular fractures, but was widely believed to carry significant systemic risks. Current experience suggests that effective medical management can minimize these risks, and that skeletal traction is a viable alternative to surgery, though with slightly impaired function and a prolonged, costly hospital stay. However, because skeletal traction offers no significant benefit for the majority of ambulatory patients, surgical treatment is the well-accepted norm.[8]

The timing of surgical treatment deserves special consideration. Urgent stabilization of femoral fractures has been recognized as beneficial for healthy young patients with high-energy injuries. This is not as clear for the elderly, who may have significant associated medical problems. Preoperative diagnosis and management should focus on physiologic derangements that increase risks of mortality and morbidity. If these can be corrected, in whole or in part, surgery becomes safer. Because of this, it is generally believed that surgery should be delayed long enough for diagnosis and urgent medical management. However, delay beyond this is unlikely to help the patient, and offers no additional benefit. Moreover, delaying surgery does increase cost by adding to length of hospitalization. Thus, the current diagnosis-related group-based reimbursement system and the economics of hospital care provide additional pressures for early surgery, as soon as the patient's condition permits. In some hospitals, operating room availability for such urgent, but nonemergent, procedures is limited. Performing hip fracture surgery unnecessarily late at night because of insufficient operating room space and staff may increase risk of complications and interfere with management.

Regional Surgical Concerns

Intertrochanteric Fractures

The mechanical challenge of hip fracture fixation is to create a composite of bone and fixation device that maintains satisfactory alignment until the bone has healed securely. For any patient, fracture configuration and bone quality are arbitrary; the surgeon can only control how the fragments are reassembled (the reduction), which device is chosen, and the location and technique of its application. Although the radiographically obvious fixation device may appear to be the most significant part of the process, proper fracture alignment and correct insertion of the fixation device are much more important.

An error in either will lead to fixation failure despite the strongest implant. Successful fixation involves (1) a reduction that allows the bone to carry a significant share of the load across the fracture zone; (2) placing the fixation device centrally in the femoral head where the bone density is greatest; and (3) attaching it securely distally. When these tasks are accomplished, surprisingly flimsy devices can maintain alignment until the fracture is healed.

A number of different implants have been developed for intertrochanteric fractures. The sliding hip screw (compression hip screw) has become the most commonly used, and is generally regarded as the most reliable type of device for extracapsular fractures. It has a large proximally threaded screw inserted into the femoral head and a lateral plate with a sleeve that fits over the shaft of the screw, maintaining a predetermined angle between screw and plate (generally 135° to 150°). The plates come in different lengths, and are attached to the lateral aspect of the femoral shaft, typically with four screws below the fracture site. Telescoping of the two parts allows the fracture fragments to impact, and thus increases the likelihood that they will bear weight, rather than transferring it to an implant that holds them apart and risks failure with repetitive loading. The screw is cannulated for insertion over a guide wire. This reduces the risk of incorrect placement. Improvements in metallurgy and design have increased the resistance of these devices to fatigue failure, which is now limited to rare cases of nonunion. Should fixation failure occur, it is usually because of the device penetrating the bone proximally, screw breakage, or pull-out distally. These events are rare and occur only when the limit of telescoping has been reached, so that the screw threads rest on the sleeve of the side plate, transferring all load from the femoral head through the implant. A number of variations have been proposed in the basic design of these implants, but these are relatively minor, such as more durable metals, surface texture, and design of proximal screw.

Other fixation devices designed for this region also deserve mention. Older, one-piece implants composed of a nail with attached side-plate (such as the Jewett nail), have generally been supplanted by the hip compression screw, which has less risk of device failure or cut-out, and places less stringent demands on achieving a fracture reduction that provides immediate loadsharing. Certain fracture patterns, such as the reverse-oblique, are prone to significant displacement after fixation with a sliding hip screw. An implant that prevents displacement may be advantageous for such fractures, in spite of its exposure to increased loading. Ninety-five degree blade-plates or screw-plates, more typically used for the distal femur, fill this role satisfactorily, but device breakage is a possibility unless fracture healing occurs before metal fatigue.

Intramedullary devices lie closer to the vector of weightbearing forces across the hip. Therefore, they offer the theoretical benefit of being exposed to lower bending moments. Any intramedullary device for this region must gain secure purchase in the proximal (head and neck) femoral fragment. Two basic approaches have been attempted. In the first, a two-part implant is used, with one part directed into the head and neck, and the other placed along the femoral shaft from the greater trochanteric region distally. Examples are the Kuntscher Y-nail, the Zickel nail, the recently developed gamma nail, and the so-called reconstruction nail, which extends the full length of the femoral shaft with holes for distal locking screws, and for two proximally directed femoral head screws. The second approach to intramedullary fixation of extracapsular hip fractures involves so-called condylocephalic implants, inserted through distal entry portals at or just above the femoral condyles, and curved to enter and transfix the femoral head. An early Kuntscher prototype, Ender nails, and the Harris nail are examples of this concept. Nearly any implant that is correctly inserted has a high likelihood of successfully fixing a properly reduced, *stable* intertrochanteric fracture.

Kyle and associates[9] reviewed their results with intertrochanteric fractures and found that complications were rare in noncomminuted fractures treated with sliding hip devices. Similar good results were noted in comminuted intertrochanteric fractures, unless significant comminution extended into the subtrochanteric region. A later review of such subtrochanteric-intertrochanteric fractures in which durable sliding screws were used showed that fixation failures were limited to elderly osteoporotic patients, almost all with reverse oblique fractures.

Most comparative studies to date confirm the superiority of the modern sliding hip screw for fixation of unstable fractures. The theoretical benefits of alternative designs have not been realized clinically, sometimes because of technical problems during a surgeon's early experience with a new implant, and sometimes because of less mechanical stability of the implant or its attachments to the bone. Intramedullary devices have been particularly alluring because of their promise of "less-invasive" surgery, akin to closed intramedullary nailing for femoral shaft fractures. However, medical morbidity is not reduced by such procedures, and seems instead to be increased by less stable fixation. Additionally, fracture fixation complications are almost always more frequent with these devices.[10-14]

Well-accepted indications have not been developed for use of implants other than sliding hip screws for basilar neck and intertrochanteric fractures. Occasionally a surgeon may choose a condylocephalic device when fracture fixation is necessary, but soft-tissue problems prevent use of an incision near the hip, or in an effort to reduce the risk of fracture distal to a side plate applied to a pathologically weak femoral shaft. Very unstable fractures, such as the reverse intertrochanteric pattern or highly comminuted injuries, may be more successfully fixed with a nontelescoping implant, such as the 95° blade-plate or screw-plate, especially in younger patients for whom preservation of normal anatomic relationships might be more compatible with greater functional demands. The use of autogenous bone graft to encourage restoration of a medial weightbearing bony buttress that protects against implant failure has been advocated by some. Others urge indirect reduction with complete avoidance of surgical contact with the radial fracture zone, so that soft-tissue attachments and fracture healing are not compromised. While the gamma nail or analogous devices might similarly stabilize an anatomic reduction, clinical comparisons strongly suggest higher associated complication rates.

In addition to implant choice, a few other surgical options exist for improving the fixation of unstable intertrochanteric fractures. Unfortunately, there is little comparative data regarding their indications and results. One such option is the choice of reduction. In unstable intertrochanteric fractures, displacement can be made less likely by realigning the fracture fragments (for example, with an osteotomy) to obtain better contact between the proximal and distal fragment. Compared to sliding hip screw fixation in a nearly anatomic alignment, however, outcomes are not improved, and deformity caused by shortening or abnormal neck-shaft angles seems to correlate with unsatisfactory gait. A second option is to use bone cement along with a fixation device. Patients with significant osteoporosis and a resulting high risk of fixation device cutout may obtain additional stability when adjunctive methylmethacrylate bone cement is used. A few encouraging reports exist, but indications for this infrequently used technique remain obscure. A third option is to place restrictions on the patient's weightbearing activities, in hopes that reduced loading will allow fracture healing before mechanical failure of fixation. While this approach is basic in the care of young, cooperative patients, it may not be possible in the elderly who are often unable to limit weightbearing, even when restricted to bed and chair activities. Yet another option in the elderly osteoporotic patient is the use of hemi or total hip replacement arthroplasty. While common and well-accepted for treatment of displaced intracapsular fractures in this population, replacement arthroplasty is rarely used for extracapsular fractures except as a salvage procedure, or when preexisting significant hip arthritis exists. Absence of an intact proximal femur mandates a special implant design. Problems with reattachment of the greater trochanter and with alignment and fixation of the femoral prosthesis have been noted. Although mechanical studies suggest that a cemented proximal femoral endoprosthesis can withstand greater load than a repaired intertrochanteric fracture, the low incidence of failure after hip screw fixation raises serious questions about the indications for arthroplasty instead of fixation of these injuries.

Complications After Fixation

Current reports of surgical treatment for intertrochanteric hip fractures indicate that fracture-related problems are rare. For example,

Larsson and associates[15] reported reoperations for wound infection (<1% with prophylactic antibiotics), technical complications with fixation (2.8%), and nonunion (0.5%). They noted 1.2% thromboembolic complications with dextran 70 prophylaxis. Only 80% of their ambulatory patients regained the same level of function. One-year mortality was 18%. The increased morbidity and mortality are apparently independent of fracture fixation. While functional ability is often less than before injury, it is rarely possible to relate the increased disability to fracture alignment and healing. Medical, cognitive, and psychosocial problems are far more important, and appear to set limitations that cannot be overcome by foreseeable improvements in fracture care.

Opportunities for Improving Results

When careful analysis of fracture fixation failures is carried out, it appears that most involve technical errors, primarily inappropriate reductions, and/or misplaced fixation devices. It would thus seem that efforts to decrease the frequency of fracture complications would be better directed toward improvements in surgical technique, instead of newer implants. Aspects to consider include intraoperative fluoroscopy and fracture tables, surgical instruments, and improved simulations for teaching and practicing fracture fixation.

Perhaps even more significant will be the understanding that comes from improved studies of clinical results. These require more precise descriptions of patients and their injuries, especially in terms of preoperative function and medical conditions, osteoporosis (bone density and related structural characteristics), and fracture pattern. Given that sliding hip screw fixation of an "anatomically aligned" fracture is the current standard, with usually acceptable results, those relatively few patients in whom it is not likely to succeed must be identified, and then the reasons for failure must be analyzed before proposing solutions. Unfortunately, orthopaedic tradition is one of introducing new fixation devices, rather than clarifying the application of existing tools.

Although there seems to be relatively little room for significant improvement in healing of intertrochanteric fractures, fruitful opportunities exist for better outcomes from attention to comprehensive rehabilitation, as previously discussed. Valuable studies will properly define and stratify patient characteristics, and prospectively compare medical and rehabilitative management techniques, while comprehensively evaluating functional outcome. To ensure widest applicability, multicenter, community-based studies will be required. In the end, the ultimate justification for any treatment protocol must be the results it achieves. To date, studies comparing alternative treatments do not truly report outcome, but look at only a few parameters in small, selected groups of patients. Recognizing that there are limits on the resources that can be devoted to health care, valid information is needed about all of the costs of alternative treatments, including those resulting from long-term care, and about management of complications. Only then can therapeutic decisions based on informed cost-effectiveness analyses be made.

Subtrochanteric Fractures

As previously mentioned, subtrochanteric fractures initially received separate recognition as a category of extracapsular hip fractures with poorer results after surgery. Indeed, early results were so poor that some surgeons recommended that these fractures be treated non-surgically, with prolonged skeletal traction, and cumbersome cast-braces. Improved surgical results have led to the general agreement that essentially all subtrochanteric fractures are best treated with surgical fixation. [16,17]

Several classifications have been proposed, but now that locked intramedullary nails have been shown to provide reliable control for more distal subtrochanteric fractures, independent of their location or fracture pattern, the important aspects of these injuries relate to the integrity of the nail insertion site (piriformis fossa) and to which configuration of proximal locking screw is required—angled distally into the region of the lesser trochanter (centromedullary), or angled proximally into the femoral head (cephalomedullary), when comminution precludes use of the distal site. Such a consideration of treatment alternatives results in a classification similar to that proposed by Russell and Taylor[17] with four categories of subtrochanteric fracture: IA, piriformis fossa and lesser trochanter intact; IB, piriformis fossa intact with lesser trochanteric comminution; IIA, piriformis fossa involved, lesser trochanteric region intact; and IIB, both piriformis fossa and lesser trochanter involved. It is also important to recognize the two distinct categories of patients who sustain subtrochanteric fractures: younger individuals with high-energy injuries to normal bone and older individuals with fractures of osteoporotic bone. The former require attention to all the potential problems of the multiply injured; the latter may have more problems with fracture fixation. Future studies of subtrochanteric fracture treatment should analyze separately these two groups of patients.

Several important questions about subtrochanteric fractures remain to be resolved. While some surgeons do not use intramedullary nails for fixation of these fractures when the nail entry site is involved, others have reported satisfactory results in such cases. Better guidelines are needed for choosing among cephalomedullary (reconstruction-type) nails, 95° blade-plate or screw-plate devices, and sliding hip screws. Although cephalomedullary nails appear promising for selected high-energy subtrochanteric fractures, their results in elderly patients with osteoporosis are not as well documented.

Medial bone grafting has often been suggested when subtrochanteric fractures are treated with open reduction and internal fixation with either of the latter two implant categories. It now appears that so-called indirect reduction techniques can achieve similar results, just as seen routinely with closed intramedullary nailing. These involve preservation of bone fragment vascularity (soft-tissue attachments) and use of fixation that permits enough fracture site mobility to avoid inhibiting callus formation. More information is needed about the indications for bone grafting of subtrochanteric fractures, as well as indications and optimal techniques and implants for indirect reduction methods.

Summary and Conclusions

For patients with extracapsular fractures, fracture healing is rarely a problem, and modern fixation techniques reliably permit ambulatory treatment. Nonetheless, opportunities for improving outcome may be found in better overall patient management and rehabilitation, and in reducing technical errors, the most common cause of infrequent fracture-site complications. Community-based outcome studies, with appropriate stratification of patients, are sorely needed to define optimal managment of these injuries. Such studies should take precedence over development of new fracture fixation devices.

References

1. Mullen JO, Mullen NL: Hip fracture mortality: A prospective, multifactorial study to predict and minimize death risk. *Clin Orthop* 1992;280:214-222.
2. Evans EM: The treatment of trochanteric fractures of the femur. *J Bone Joint Surg* 1949;31B;190-203.
3. Zuckerman JD, Schon LC: Hip fractures, in Zuckerman JD (ed): *Comprehensive Care of Orthopaedic Injuries in the Elderly*. Baltimore, MD, Urban & Schwarzenberg, 1990, chap 3, pp 23-111.
4. Zuckerman JD, Sakales SR, Fabian DR, et al: Hip fractures in geriatric patients: Results of an interdisciplinary hospital care program. *Clin Orthop* 1992;274:213-225.
5. Levy RN, Capozzi JD, Mont MA: Intertrochanteric hip fractures, in Browner BD, Jupiter JB, Levine AM (eds): *Skeletal Trauma: Fractures, Dislocations, Ligamentous Injuries*. Philadelphia, PA, WB Saunders, 1992, vol 2, chap 44, pp 1442-1484.
6. Strain JJ, Lyons JS, Hammer JS, et al: Cost offset from a psychiatric consultation-liaison intervention with elderly hip fracture patients. *Am J Psychiatr* 1991;148:1044-1049.
7. Walheim G, Barrios C, Stark A, et al: Postoperative improvement of walking capacity in patients with trochanteric hip fracture: A prospective analysis 3 and 6 months after surgery. *J Orthop Trauma* 1990;4:137-143.
8. Parker MJ, Myles JW, Anand JK, et al: Cost-benefit analysis of hip fracture treatment. *J Bone Joint Surg* 1992;74B:261-264.
9. Kyle RF, Gustilo RB, Premer RF: Analysis of six hundred and twenty-two intertrochanteric hip fractures. *J Bone Joint Surg* 1979;61A:216-221.
10. Ekeland A, Aune AK, Odegaard B, et al: Complications after gamma nailing of proximal femoral fractures. Presented at the Sixtieth Annual Meeting of the American Academy of Orthopaedic Surgeons, San Francisco, CA, Feb 22, 1993.

11. Goldhagen P, O'Connor DR, Schwartz EG, et al: A prospective comparative study of the compression hip screw and the gamma nail. Presented at the Sixtieth Annual Meeting of the American Academy of Orthopaedic Surgeons, San Francisco, CA, Feb 22, 1993.

12. Hogh J, Andersen KS, Duus B, et al: Gamma nail vs. DHS in the treatment of trochanteric and subtrochanteric fractures. Presented at the Sixtieth Annual Meeting of the American Academy of Orthopaedic Surgeons, Feb 22, 1993.

13. Mott M, Kronick JL, Fitzgerald RH Jr, et al: Gamma nail versus the sliding hip screw. a prospective randomized comparison. Presented at the Sixtieth Annual Meeting of the American Academy of Orthopaedic Surgeons, Feb 22, 1993.

14. Nungu S, Olerud C, Rehnberg L: Treatment of intertrochanteric fractures: Comparison of Ender nails and sliding screw plates. *J Orthop Trauma* 1991;5:452-457.

15. Larsson S, Friberg S, Hansson LI: Trochanteric fractures: Mobility, complications, and mortality in 607 cases treated with the sliding-screw technique. *Clin Orthop* 1990;260:232-241.

16. Alho A, Ekeland A, Stromsoe K: Subtrochanteric femoral fractures treated with locked intramedullary nails: Experience from 31 cases. *Acta Orthop Scand* 1991;62:573-576.

17. Russell TA, Taylor JC: Subtrochanteric fractures of the femur, in Browner BD, Jupiter JB, Levine AM, et al (eds): *Skeletal Trauma: Fractures, Dislocations, Ligamentous Injuries*. Philadelphia, PA, WB Saunders, 1992, vol 2, chap 45, pp 1485-1524.

Section Four

Prevention

Chapter 10

Risk Factors and Opportunities for Prevention of Falls in the Frail Elderly

Lewis A. Lipsitz, MD

Background

Falls are a common source of serious morbidity and mortality in the elderly, often resulting in loss of independent function and the need for institutionalized care. Falls occur annually in 35% to 40% of community-dwelling elderly, and in as many as 50% of elderly patients receiving institutionalized care. Fortunately, most falls do not result in injury, but 6% are associated with fractures. In the United States, over 250,000 hip fractures each year are a result of falls alone.[1]

Several factors increase the risk of falls among older individuals. First, there are age-related changes that impair postural stability and blood pressure homeostasis, making older persons more vulnerable to falls and syncope. These changes include the loss of proprioceptive sensory receptors, afferent fibers, and central nervous system neurons in the frontal cortex, basal ganglia, and cerebellum—resulting in a stiff, parkinsonian gait and increased body sway; as well as decreased baroreflex sensitivity, reduced renal salt and water conservation, and impaired ventricular diastolic filling—all predisposing elderly people to hypotension.[1] Second, in addition to the age-related changes, disease-related factors such as arthritis, cardiovascular disease, and visual impairment further increase risk of falls. As a result of the development of disease, the elderly often adopt a sedentary lifestyle, become deconditioned, and have difficulty adapting to environmental stress. Therefore, environmental hazards that may be easily overcome by more agile, younger individuals often precipitate falls in the elderly. Finally, iatrogenic factors, such as the use of medications or improperly used assistive devices, may further increase the risk of falling. Commonly used anticholinergic medications are particularly hazardous, including antihistamines, antidepressants, antipsychotics, and sedatives. Possible side effects from medication, including impaired alertness, postural instability, or hypotension (related to syncope), contribute to an increased risk of falling.

Risk Factors for Falls in the Frail Elderly

In order to target those individuals at greatest risk and design appropriate intervention strategies, several previous studies have attempted to define risk factors for falls in various populations. In four prospective community-dwelling populations studied to date,[2-5] several common risk factors have been identified. Dementia has been identified as a risk factor for falls in two studies. Possible side effects attributed to psychotropic medications were an important risk factor in one study and were associated with falls in women in another. Arthritis and lower extremity weakness were found as risk factors in all four investigations. Impaired ability to rise from a chair without using the arms to push off was also found in two studies, one of which showed an association with falls only in men. Gait and balance problems also were significantly related to falls in four of the studies, and multiple factors were found to compound the risk in at least two investigations (Table 1).

There have been relatively few studies of factors associated with falls in patients receiving institutionalized care, despite the fact that this is a population at highest risk of serious consequences from falls. Nursing home residents are more likely to have multiple factors contributing to falls.[6]

To determine causes and clinical correlates of recurrent falls in ambulatory, frail, elderly patients, 70 recurrent fallers and 56 nonfallers (mean age = 87 years) from two long-term care facilities were evaluated,[7] including a detailed history, physical examination, performance-oriented mobility assessment, and laboratory studies. Primary causes of falls, including stroke, parkinsonism, blindness, drug-related hypotension, and arthritis, were established for the most recent falls in 51 (73%) fallers. Eighteen fallers (26%) had multiple conditions that could not be prioritized for their contribution to the fall. Fallers were more often women, had more functional impairment, and were taking more medications than nonfallers. Specific diseases did not distinguish fallers from nonfallers. Fallers of both sexes took more steps to make a 360-degree turn, could not rise from a chair without pushing off, had a higher prevalence of antidepressant use, and had an impaired sense of position in the toes. These easily obtained clinical variables characterized nearly three fourths of ambulatory elderly nursing home residents with a history of recurrent falls.

This study highlighted hypotension and muscle weakness, two areas that were particularly amenable to intervention.

Hypotensive Causes of Falls

To determine whether transient hypotension in response to common daily activities, including medication ingestion, may be one of the many factors contributing to the high prevalence of falls among the

Table 1 Independent predictors of falls common to case-controlled studies of community-dwelling elderly people (older than 60 years)

	Study			
Predictors	Campbell 1989 (N = 761)	Nevitt* 1989 (N = 325)	Robbins 1989 (N = 68)	Tinetti 1988 (N = 336)
	Adjusted Odds Ratio†			
Dementia			+	5.0
Psychotropics	1.6 (female)			28.3
Arthritis/leg weakness	1.8-2.7	2.7	+	3.8
Chair stand	3.4 (male)	3.0		
Gait and balance problem	1.7-2.6 (sway)	2.7 (tandem)	+	1.0-1.9
Multiple risks		+	+	

*Recurrent, nonsyncopal falls.
†If no odds ratio is reported, the plus sign indicates that these predictors had a statistically significant association with falls.

elderly, blood pressure and heart rate responses to a standardized series of activities were examined in 38 institutionalized fallers (87 ± 6 years), 20 institutionalized nonfallers (85 ± 5 years), and 10 healthy, young control subjects (24 ± 3 years).[8] The coefficient of variation for systolic blood pressure during all activities was higher in elderly subjects than in young control subjects. In contrast, the coefficient of variation for heart rate during all activities was higher in young subjects than in elderly subjects, demonstrating impaired baroreflex responses to blood pressure changes in old age. Nursing home residents had marked blood pressure reduction following meals and administration of nitroglycerin. This reduction was significantly greater in fallers than nonfallers, independent of the cause of the fall. Thus, institutionalized elderly people have marked blood pressure variability and hypotensive responses following meals and administration of nitroglycerin. A decline in blood pressure during these common preloading-reducing stresses may predispose some elderly people to falls. Furthermore, behavioral changes such as lying down after meals or separating medication administration from meal ingestion might be important interventions to prevent falls in this frail population.

Muscle Weakness

Several studies indicate that various measures of muscle strength, including the chair stand, which evaluates extensors of the knee (quadriceps) and hip (gluteus), have been found to be associated with falls.[3,4]

In addition, there are direct correlations between muscle strength (measured as leg extensor power[9] or the one repetition maximum of the quadriceps muscles[10]) and various functional measures such as walking speed, stair climbing speed, and chair rising speed, all of which are intermediary variables associated with falls risk. These observations have led to the following research questions: (1) Is it possible to increase muscle strength among frail elderly fallers through a program of high-intensity resistance training? (2) Does an increase in quadriceps muscle strength improve functional gait characteristics that are associated with falls risk?

The first question was investigated in a pilot study of ten elderly nursing home residents, mean age 90 ± 1 years, who participated in an eight-week program of resistance training of the leg quadriceps muscles.[10] This project, directed by Dr. Maria Fiatarone at the Hebrew Rehabilitation Center for Aged in Boston, Massachusetts, demonstrated significant gains in the one repetition maximum of both legs after eight weeks of training. On average, the nine subjects who completed training gained $174\% \pm 31\%$ (mean $\pm$ SEM) in their one repetition maximum in both legs. In addition, there was a significant increase in quadriceps and hamstring muscle area on CT scans following this training program. In total, there was a $9\% \pm 4.5\%$ change in midthigh muscle area attributable to training.

In response to these preliminary data, Dr. Fiatarone is currently directing a prospective, placebo-controlled randomized trial of resistance training, nutritional supplementation, and both in 100 elderly residents of the Hebrew Rehabilitation Center for Aged. This study will address the second question posed, to determine the effect of muscle strengthening and/or nutritional supplementation on functional mobility. Whether this will result in improved functional capacity, and ultimately, a reduction in the rate of falls, cannot be determined until the trial is completed.

Opportunities for Preventing Falls in the Elderly

Based on currently available data, there are at least five factors that are associated with the development of falls in the frail elderly, and are potentially modifiable through readily available interventions. These factors include: (1) muscle weakness, which can be improved through resistance exercise training; (2) effects of psychotropic medications, which often can be discontinued, reduced in dose, or replaced by other medications; (3) hypotension, which may improve following discontinuation of medications, volume expansion, or simple behavioral therapies to avoid hypotensive stresses; (4) impaired balance, which may be improved by balance training or footwear and assistive devices that provide a wide base of support; and (5) environmental hazards, which can be eliminated or better compensated for by improving visual acuity. Interventions such as cataract removal, corrective lenses, or increased lighting can help the elderly better adapt visually to potential environmental hazards.

Many of these modifiable risk factors are readily identifiable in the nursing home population, particularly with widespread use of the new Health Care Financing Administration-mandated Resident Assessment Instrument that is being used in all Medicare- and Medicaid-supported nursing homes throughout the United States.[11] This instrument provides critical information (called the Minimum Data Set) that can be used to target at-risk individuals. Future studies are needed to determine the impact of the interventions previously suggested on preventing falls in the elderly.

Conclusions

In summary, there are several important age- and disease-related factors that make the elderly vulnerable to falling, together with the adverse effects of a sedentary lifestyle, attendant muscle weakness, and medications that have sedating and hypotensive side effects. Each of these factors is potentially modifiable. An intensive program of resistance exercises can improve quadriceps muscle strength, and weakness of the quadriceps muscle is associated with impairments in gait that increase the risk of falling. Future investigations of resistance training and other interventions should prove effective in reversing the multiple risk factors for falls in the frail elderly.

References

1. Lipsitz LA: Falls in the elderly, in Kelley WN, DeVita VT Jr, DuPont HL, et al (eds): *Textbook of Internal Medicine*, ed 2. Philadelphia, PA, JB Lippincott, 1992, chap 522, vol 2, pp 2420-2423.
2. Tinetti ME, Speechley M, Ginter SF: Risk factors for falls among elderly persons living in the community. *N Engl J Med* 1988;319:1701-1707.
3. Campbell AJ, Borrie MJ, Spears GF: Risk factors for falls in a community-based prospective study of people 70 years and older. *J Gerontol* 1989;44:M112-M117.
4. Nevitt MC, Cummings SR, Kidd S, et al: Risk factors for recurrent nonsyncopal falls: A prospective study. *JAMA* 1989;261:2663-2668.
5. Robbins AS, Rubenstein LZ, Josephson KR, et al: Predictors of falls among elderly people: Results of two population-based studies. *Arch Intern Med* 1989;149: 1628-1633.
6. Tinetti ME, Williams TF, Mayewski R: Fall risk index for elderly patients based on number of chronic disabilities. *Am J Med* 1986;80:429-434.
7. Lipsitz LA, Jonsson PV, Kelley MM, et al: Causes and correlates of recurrent falls in ambulatory frail elderly. *J Gerontol* 1991;46:M114-M122.
8. Jonsson PV, Lipsitz LA, Kelley M, et al: Hypotensive responses to common daily activities in institutionalized elderly: A potential risk for recurrent falls. *Arch Intern Med* 1990;150:1518-1524.
9. Bassey EJ, Fiatarone MA, O'Neill EF, et al: Leg extensor power and functional performance in very old men and women. *Clin Sci* 1992;82:321-327.
10. Fiatarone MA, Marks EC, Ryan ND, et al: High-intensity strength training in nonagenarians: Effects on skeletal muscle. *JAMA* 1990;263:3029-3034.
11. Morris JN, Hawes C, Fries BE, et al: Designing the national resident assessment institute for nursing homes. *Gerontologist* 1990;30:293-307.

Chapter 11

Geriatric Falls Program Development at the Hospital for Joint Diseases

Joseph D. Zuckerman, MD
Adam Karp, MD
Janet Weinstein, RN, NP
Jane Potts, CSW

Falls are a major health hazard for the elderly. Not only are falls the sixth leading cause of death in persons over the age of 65, but one fall in 20 results in a hip fracture. Falls are also an important indicator of a decline in functional status and should lead to careful assessment of possible contributing factors, which would include a systemic evaluation for underlying diseases, and a study of medications, gait and balance, and environmental risks. Approximately 90% of falls do not result in serious injury, but may still have important consequences. Many elderly limit their level of activity after a fall. This reduction in activity can result in a steady loss of functional status.[1-6]

A Geriatric Falls Program was developed at the Hospital for Joint Diseases in New York to learn as much as possible about the circumstances and outcomes of falls by the elderly, to help them more adequately address their fears of falling, and ultimately to prevent further falls and alterations in older adults' lifestyles. It is hoped that this program will serve as a pilot in the development of strategies to treat the older person who falls. During the first two years of this project, data will be collected on the older people seen in the unit. Their progress will be evaluated, and we will determine whether quality of life improves after evaluation and whether these people injure themselves less than historic controls. The program has three components: education and outreach, outpatient evaluation, and inpatient evaluation.

Education and Outreach

The education and outreach component consists of a community education program directed at home-dwelling elderly living in an urban setting as well as organizations servicing the elderly. A team approach is used, consisting of a geriatrician, geriatric nurse practitioner, and social worker. The geriatrician focuses on medical problems and medication usage; the nurse practitioner talks about home and street safety and shoewear; and the social worker discusses available community resources. At the conclusion of the educational program, information is given on who is appropriate for the Geriatric Falls Program, how to schedule an evaluation, and what can be offered through the interdisciplinary team at the Hospital for Joint Diseases.

Organizations servicing the elderly are identified by the geriatric nurse practitioner and the social worker. Information about the Geriatric Falls Program is provided to organizations throughout Manhattan via the Manhattan Boroughwide Interagency Council on Aging, Inc., which is composed of organizations that serve the elderly and are responsive to their problems. Further contact with the member organizations and the scheduling of education outreach talks continues, with the social worker contacting each agency, scheduling talks, and providing information for referral. In addition, the social worker is contacted by private home care organizations, city programs serving the elderly, and privately funded volunteer organizations serving the elderly. These groups all have requested additional information about referrals to the Falls Evaluation Unit and have expressed their desire to participate in the education and outreach component. For these groups a different type of program designed for health care professionals involved in the care of the elderly is presented by the team.

The geriatrician describes the medical aspects of falls evaluation and treatment, beginning the presentation with an introduction to the field of geriatrics and general aspects of well-being of the older person. The interview process, during which the caregiver tries to determine the cause of a person's gait abnormality, is described. Medication in the elderly is stressed, with a description of how some drugs, such as long-acting benzodiazepines and hypotensive agents, may cause falling. In addition, the role of alcohol and alcoholism in the elderly and its relationship to falls is discussed.

The geriatrician also focuses on specific aspects of the physical examination that are critical to the evaluation of the elderly person who falls. A complete eye examination, a hearing evaluation, and a musculoskeletal examination specifically directed to the lower extremities are important. A review of good foot care and shoe selection, crucial aspects of mobility sometimes overlooked by the primary care physician, are discussed. The geriatrician also considers some laboratory evaluations that may be useful in the older person who falls, emphasizing the importance of thyroid evaluation, B12 and folate levels, and screening for syphilis.

The geriatric nurse practitioner then conducts an open discussion, advising on how to make the home safe. Questions and comments are encouraged. During the presentation, a checklist of suggested home improvements for stairways, hallways, bathrooms, and bedrooms is provided to the participants. The geriatric nurse practitioner exhibits safety devices, such as bathroom grab bars, reachers, nonskid tape, and reflective tape, and discusses how these items can be obtained. The geriatric nurse practitioner also addresses hazards outside the home. The use of shopping carts, public transportation, and the often treacherous task of ambulating on the streets of New York City are also discussion topics. This discussion emphasizes the changes that the older adult must make to insure safety and mobility, considering that as many as half of all fall-related injuries could be prevented by simple modifications in the home environment.

The social worker's presentation focuses on a case example used to illustrate the manner in which counseling services are provided to older people. The example includes work with family members to strengthen relationships and referral to community programs to address special needs and provide socialization. The social worker educates older people and their families about home-care programs, subsidized community services, and entitlement programs that provide an opportunity for change and an improved quality of life. Through the Geriatric Falls Program, the social worker can offer counseling on an outpatient basis and enlist the help of support groups when indicated. By addressing each individual's needs, the social worker devises a coherent plan that insures continuity of care. Following the outreach talk, the social worker acts as a liaison with the community organization to answer questions and encourage referrals for the Geriatric Falls Evaluation Unit.

Outpatient Evaluation Unit

The Falls Evaluation Unit is for older people who have fallen and whose fear of falling has disrupted their quality of life. Once an appointment is made, the unit secretary sends out a letter describing the evaluation process. A questionnaire with a falls diary is included with the letter to facilitate obtaining a medical history. Two days before the visit, the geriatric nurse practitioner contacts the patient to address any questions or concerns.

On the day of the visit, the patient is seen by an interdisciplinary team that includes the geriatrician, geriatric nurse practitioner, and social worker. The geriatric nurse practitioner, under the supervision of the geriatrician, performs a comprehensive assessment. The evaluation includes an in-depth history, including a falls history, medical (including information about medications and allergies) and surgical history, and social history. Next, a thorough physical examination is performed, with major emphasis on gait and balance.[7] The patient is also observed ambulating over a long distance to evaluate if changes in gait may contribute to falls. Neurologic disorders, visual changes or impairment, vestibular dysfunction, decreased muscle strength in the lower extremities, foot disorders, or acute problems that might contribute to falls, such as orthostatic hypotension, congestive heart failure, or pneumonia, are also evaluated. All medication is reviewed for its appropriateness.

The social work assessment is provided for patients believed to be at risk based on the Geriatric Falls Program High Risk Screen, which focuses on different psychosocial issues. When interviewing the patient, the social worker distinguishes needs relevant to daily functioning and home management, the degree and extent of formal and informal supports, and the presenting problem. Using the identified needs, the social worker forms a plan and discusses the identified goals and objectives with the patient. The social worker provides educational information, referral for community services, and interventions appropriate to the individual situation. Where applicable, outpatient counseling and support groups are offered.

Once all the information is obtained, the interdisciplinary team reviews the findings and determines a treatment plan. The treatment recommendations are generally oriented toward preventing additional falls and allowing the patient to continue to maintain an independent lifestyle. Specialist evaluations, in the areas of neurology, cardiology, and physiatry, when needed, are scheduled for the follow-up visit; during this time, the pediatric nurse practitioner is the primary contact with the patient and coordinates all the necessary specialist evaluations.

To assure continuity of care, the social worker functions as a liaison between the referring community organization and the Geriatric Falls Program. The geriatrician and the nurse practitioner summarize the medical treatment plan in a letter to the referring physician or community organization.

Additional outreach and education will be provided through support groups offered by the geriatric nurse practitioner and the social worker for people who have been evaluated in the outpatient unit. Support groups provide the opportunity for mutual support by identifying the impact of falls or fear of falls, and the impact of isolation on daily life. Education and instruction in body mechanics and movement exercises offer methods for coping with physical limitations. Discussion of community resources and alternative programs offers additional opportunity for self-development and socialization. These opportunities will be offered to Geriatric Falls Program patients as well as to members of community organizations.

Finally, for follow-up purposes, patients are contacted every month by the geriatric nurse practitioner to monitor their progress and determine if further evaluation is needed.

Inpatient Evaluation

Another component of the Falls Evaluation Unit is the identification and treatment of older persons who present to the Hospital for Joint

Diseases for orthopaedic injuries resulting from falls. Every person who arrives at the Urgent Orthopaedic Care Center or is admitted to the hospital with a falls-related diagnosis and is over the age of 65 is referred to the geriatric nurse practitioner for evaluation. The geriatric nurse practitioner screens every patient in person, or by telephone if they are no longer in the hospital. These findings are then reviewed, and further work-up and evaluation is decided on. These efforts are coordinated with the orthopaedic surgeon and medical consultant involved in the case.

This system allows admitted patients to be clustered on one floor in the hospital. An interdisciplinary meeting including the geriatrician, geriatric nurse practitioner, nurse in charge of the floor, social worker, dietician, and physical therapist is held weekly, during which the inpatients are discussed and further management is coordinated.

The primary goal of the Geriatric Falls Program at the Hospital for Joint Diseases is to improve the quality of life and the health of the older adult by providing a careful assessment of the medications, diseases, and psychosocial factors that may increase their risk of falls. With the interdisciplinary team's understanding of the cause of these falls, older adults may be able to function more independently and resume a normal standard of life following a fall.

References

1. Duthie EH Jr: Falls. *Med Clin North Am* 1989;73:1321-1336.
2. Hindmarsh JJ, Estes EH Jr: Falls in older persons: Causes and interventions. *Arch Intern Med* 1989;149:2217-2222.
3. Nevitt MC, Cummings SR, Kidd S, et al: Risk factors for recurrent nonsyncopal falls: A prospective study. *JAMA* 1989;261:2663-2668.
4. Rubenstein LZ, Robbins AS, Josephson KR, et al: The value of assessing falls in an elderly population: A randomized clinical trial. *Ann Intern Med* 1990;113:308-316.
5. Sudarsky L: Geriatrics: Gait disorders in the elderly. *N Engl J Med* 1990;322:1441-1446.
6. Tinetti ME, Speechley M: Prevention of falls among the elderly. *N Engl J Med* 1989;320:1055-1059.
7. Tinetti ME: Performance-oriented assessment of mobility problems in elderly patients. *J Am Geriatr Soc* 1986;34:119-126.

Chapter 12

Exploring Novel Interventions to Reduce Falls in Older Individuals

Steven L. Wolf, PhD, FAPTA

Introduction

In 1990, the National Institute on Aging, in collaboration with the National Center for Nursing Research, funded a series of collaborative studies, titled Frailty and Injuries: Cooperative Studies on Intervention Techniques (FICSIT). These studies were designed to reduce frailty and improve the prospects for maintaining postural stability. Emory University in Atlanta was one of the eight sites engaged in this project. Each site devised some unique interventions, the benefits from which are now being analyzed. This presentation highlights two such interventions, computerized balance training and Tai Chi Quan. These exercise forms are diverse in their cultural origins, interfaces, and targeted training goals.

Balance Using Feedback

Over the past 17 years, physiologic feedback mechanisms have been pursued using position, force, and muscle feedback for movement control among a variety of older individuals who have had strokes, joint replacements, or amputations.[1-5]

The FICSIT trials focused on determining whether relatively sophisticated instruments that provide information about center of mass dispersion might be used constructively to change people's ability to control their center of mass when perturbed while standing on a movable platform. Up until this time, most of the work published using force feedback had involved the use of transducers or force plates.[6-8] Studies over several years had used feedback of force distribution during limb loading to examine the training of amputees to bear weight through their prostheses, in an effort to facilitate their acceptance of these devices.[9,10]

It seemed reasonable for several companies to develop devices that provide very sophisticated information about balance performance. One such device, the Balance System (Chattecx Company, Chattanooga, TN), was used in the FICSIT trial. Individuals stand on two series of forced transducers separately placed on a movable platform. A cursor appears on the screen of a monitor, giving information about the resolution of all the forces through those force plates. The cursor, in turn, can be oriented toward an individual or array of targets also placed on the screen. The goal of the individual is to move the center of mass toward the target; in other words, bring the cursor into the target range wherever the target is placed. In addition, the actual floor upon which the force plates are placed can be moved so that not only is the person trying to shift the center of mass but the standing platform can be perturbed simultaneously either in linear (anterior-posterior) or in angular (toes-up, toes-down) directions. Between platform movement and target relocations, the possible combinations and permutations become fairly sophisticated in a relatively short period.

Tai Chi

Not only do a lot of people in Eastern cultures practice Tai Chi as a martial arts form, for which it was originally intended, but many older individuals practice it as an exercise form. According to the literature,[11] Tai Chi has been practiced by older Chinese for well over 300 years, presumably because of the remediative (curative or rehabilitative) or preventive elements of Tai Chi. Most Tai Chi exercises are multiplexed forms. In Tai Chi Quan, for example, there are 108 forms. These forms are progressive sequences of more and more difficult maneuvers until body weight is controlled during rotatory trunk movements on single limb support. The sequencing becomes exceptionally sophisticated.

It was also assumed that these forms were used to correct for changes in movement that occur during the aging process—movements become slowed, trunk range of motion becomes more limited, and strength is reduced. There is an increased flexed posture, and reduced rotational movements and arm swings are noted during ambulation.

Tai Chi attempts to reverse some of these limitations. Specifically, all forms of Tai Chi have in common natural body movements and the relaxed environment in which they are done. Practitioners have to concentrate simultaneously on body movements and staying alert. There is a very clear mind/body interaction. All the movements are done in a slow, smooth, progressive manner, emphasizing bilateral and eventually unilateral movements.

This description may seem somewhat trivial until this concept is applied to frail, older people who may be depressed, overmedicated, and thinking or worrying about many things. Application of Tai Chi principles simply does not permit an individual to think about anything other than body-environment interactions. Tai Chi is very difficult to practice unless the mind is focused on the body's spatial relationship and the control of body movements. In fact, among the 72 subjects who have now gone through Tai Chi Quan training, two remarkable phenomena have transpired. About half of these subjects practice Tai Chi Quan weekly, 2.5 years after completing the 15-week program. None of them had tried it before. People are readily able to demonstrate activities that they claim they couldn't do before, including a reduction in the use of assistive devices, needed because of past falls or musculoskeletal instability. Many such individuals can now dress themselves or put on shoes without assistance.

Differences Between Balance Training and Tai Chi Quan

Table 1 summarizes the specific differences between balance training and Tai Chi Quan. Balance training requires relatively sophisticated and expensive instrumentation, is undertaken individually and involves high-technology, state-of-the-art resolution of forces through multiplexed forced transducers to yield a center of mass that is displayed on a monitor as a moving cursor. On the other hand, Tai Chi Quan is usually performed as a group activity; therefore, there is a high degree of socialization built into this activity. No equipment is required, nor is there need for special clothing. The Tai Chi Quan training can occur in any environment.

With respect to the actual mobility activities within each training paradigm, the high technology of balance feedback usually involves bilateral leg activities with the subject in a fixed position while the floor underneath is perturbed through either linear or angular displacements. On the other hand, Tai Chi Quan progresses from bilateral support to single limb support with the inclusion of slow rotatory movements that involve the trunk in combination with arm movements. Thus, individuals who progress through the "forms" of Tai Chi Quan do so by eventually narrowing the base of support and emphasizing enhanced rotational movements. This perspective is particularly intriguing because narrowed base support and rotatory movements are elements involving postural control that are often more poorly executed as a function of aging. Both balance training and Tai Chi Quan are performed in relatively quiet environments, allegedly to reduce anxiety and promote concentration.

After one week, balance training consists of a series of increasingly difficult postural demands that are introduced to subjects over the course of single sessions for each of 15 weeks. Subjects are trained to maintain the resolution of their center of mass within a target specified on the monitor directly in front of them. The training goals consist of maintaining postural stability while the platform is

Table 1 Distinct differences between computerized balance training and Tai Chi Quan

Element	Balance Training	Tai Chi Quan
Trainee	Individual	Group
Expense	High	Low
Feedback cues	External	Internal
Technology	High	Low
Mobility goals	Bilateral stance	Unilateral stance
Primary, therapeutic	Balance/trunk	Flexibility/reduced
Events	Control	Anxiety

moved in linear or angular directions. These tasks are eventually undertaken both with eyes open and with eyes closed, with the subject facing the screen or turned 90°. Full body rotation to 90° now changes the total postural demand placed on individuals as they are trained. To facilitate training under the latter condition, a second monitor is placed in front of the patients so they could still observe changes in the center of mass. Interspersed with each training session is movement of the target within a specific quadrant of the screen. Under this circumstance, the subject has to shift the center of mass within that target both under static conditions and as the platform was moved. This activity sought to stress the limits of stability. Conspicuously absent from balance training was the progressively narrowing base of support to place even further demands on postural stability.

Therapeutic Elements in Tai Chi Quan

Approximately eight components of the therapeutic basis underlying Tai Chi Quan may be of potential importance (Outline 1). However, the relation of components of Tai Chi Quan to their reputed therapeutic benefits has not been documented in the literature. Movements appear to be continuous and performed slowly. Under these circumstances, progressively greater movement is seen, the knees are flexed, and body weight shifts. For the most part, head and trunk are aligned in a straight and extended positions. Movements occur in a sequence of trunk, head, and extremity rotation. Among the 108 forms within Tai Chi Quan there appear to be asymmetrical diagonal turns in leg movements about the waist and ultimately a progression toward unilateral weightbearing. In other words, all the movement patterns usually associated with older individuals (a rounded posture, slightly flexed trunk, and limited base of support) appear to be counteracted within the components of Tai Chi Quan. Accordingly, it is interesting to speculate that the reason why older Chinese living in Eastern cultures have adopted Tai Chi as an exercise form is because the movements themselves tend to counteract postural adaptations occurring in many older, sedentary people.

Outline 1 Therapeutic elements in Tai Chi Quan

Slow movement	Diagonal turn of legs
Mind/body interactions	Weight shifting
Trunk rotation	Knee flexion/extension
Erect posture	"Feel" through feet

The Atlanta FICSIT Experience

Two hundred individuals over the age of 70 participated in the Atlanta FICSIT trial. The mean age was 76 and the ratio of women to men was 3:1. Recruitment was primarily through advertisement and word of mouth. Consequently, those individuals attracted to the FICSIT trial tended to be relatively sophisticated and active; most lived within the community and many engaged in various activities, including water aerobics. Of the 200 subjects, 72 had reported at least one or more falls in the past year. Subjects were randomly assigned to balance training (N = 64), Tai Chi Quan (N = 72), or a control group that received weekly educational discussions on topics of importance to older citizens. The dropout rate for the entire study was 16%.

Preliminary Data

One method to assess postural stability is to examine the amount of dispersion in movement under static and dynamic conditions. Specifically, the balance training and Tai Chi Quan participants were asked to stand on a balance platform with eyes open or closed and with the platform either stationary or moving. Forced transducer records were resolved in the X and Y axis of movement to determine the degree of postural sway under these conditions. Less variability in voltage-generated data points implied that subjects were more stable under each condition. Preliminary data indicate that those individuals receiving balance training showed less variability in dispersion of voltage records than those subjects undergoing Tai Chi Quan training. While on the surface these data would suggest that balance training facilitated greater postural stability, the device upon which these postural sway measures were made is identical to the training device used by the balance training group. Therefore, the possibility that reduced postural sway was caused by familiarity with the device or to a very specific learning curve cannot be dismissed.

On the other hand, the number of falls and injurious falls was substantially reduced among the Tai Chi Quan trainers, in comparison with the balance training group. This observation suggests that the components of Tai Chi Quan may actually train individuals to increase their dispersion and limits of postural stability in such a way as to help people to reduce the chance of falls under sudden perturbation conditions. This observation would explain why Tai Chi Quan trainees show greater dispersion on measuring postural stability but are better able to abort potential falls. The validity of this observation awaits further evaluation of the data. An initial review of fall behavior revealed that subjects in the balance training group had significantly greater numbers of falls than those in the Tai Chi Quan training group. In fact, 26 people in the balance training group sustained a fall, 16 of which involved injuries, with three of those injuries requiring documented medical attention. To better understand this distribution, tandem stance was examined for 10 seconds. Of the individuals assigned to the balance training group, 18 were not able to complete this balance test before the intervention. Yet these 18 people were not the same individuals who reported falls after the intervention. Therefore, the intervention cannot be considered a cause for why people fall more frequently; there is no correlation between tandem stance prior to intervention and fall behavior after the intervention among balance machine trainees.

Among the Tai Chi Quan group, 30 of 72 individuals had reported falls prior to the intervention. During the intervention there were just as many people in the Tai Chi Quan group who had reported falls as in the balance training group. After intervention, however, the falls incidence was reduced substantially, almost cut in half compared to the balance training group. With respect to injurious falls (those requiring medical attention or hospitalization), their distribution after intervention is substantially smaller than in the balance training group.

Further Assessment of Balance Training and Tai Chi Quan

There are numerous questions still being evaluated within the data set. Preliminary analysis of these data indicate that sleeping patterns and previous histories of falls may be important covariates requiring study to explain the incidence and distribution of injurious falls. The relationship between the time to the first fall and intervention assignment is also being assessed. Preliminary data analysis suggests that previous work habits, health histories, nicotine or alcohol use, and gender do not impact upon falls behavior, irrespective of an individual's assigned group.

At this point, both Tai Chi Quan participants and individuals subjected to balance training acquired varying benefits from these interventions. The Tai Chi Quan participants, upon exit interview, expressed a far more enthusiastic attitude toward their participation and a willingness to continue with this exercise form. Whether this attitude truly reflects a genuine interest in Tai Chi Quan or is precipitated by the excellent quality of training and the attitude conveyed by the Tai Chi Quan instructor is unknown. For example, when individuals participating in their particular programs were asked whether the experience had enhanced their "confidence," the Tai Chi Quan group had far more affirmative responses than the balance training group. The same pattern was apparent when participants were asked whether their normal physical activity had changed as a result of their participation in this study.

Future Perspectives

In addition to more detailed data analyses on both these interventions, there is a need to delineate more clearly the mechanisms underlying change in physiologic, functional parameters. I believe that for balance training to be an effective intervention, the limits of stability must be stressed and a progressively narrowing base of support must be incorporated into the training. Even single limb support during balance training may be an important feature to enhance postural control. In fact, I believe the dynamics of sway and the single limb support inherent in Tai Chi Quan are important components that were missing from the balance training intervention. Based on preliminary data analyses and subjective reports from all participants, I believe that progressively compromising postural stability is a necessary prerequisite to facilitating a sense of accomplishment and overcoming a fear of falling. On many occasions, Tai Chi Quan trainees commented on the number of aborted falls they experienced because they allegedly now had a strategy that could be enacted when they were suddenly perturbed. Future investigations involving balance training must incorporate repetitive experiences for participants that come as close to a real "fall" as possible.

Because of the inability to specifically relate fall occurrences to any definitive sensory or motor deficit within this sample, there is a need to explore other possibilities to account for unprecipitated falling. One logical candidate that, to date, defies description is cognitive compromise. An individual's cognition can be assessed as normal using Mini-Mental Status Examination (MMSE), yet, the individual may simply not process a visual cue normally perceived as an impending obstacle. On many occasions upon retrieving falls histories, subjects have indicated that either the obstacle "was not there" or "it was there but I didn't notice it." This possibility suggests that processing of important information may become more selective as a function of aging. If this premise proves to be true, then the mind-body interactions that are a core concept within Tai Chi Quan will prove their value because trainees will be more aware of where their bodies are spatially, even if an obstacle is not immediately perceived. Similarly, by stressing the limits of stability to the point of a "near fall," these experiences might assist individuals in responding appropriately should they actually experience an unintended fall. These interesting contributions to fall-related behavior await further analysis.

References

1. Wolf SL, Baker MP, Kelly JL: EMG biofeedback in stroke: A 1-year follow-up on the effect of patient characteristics. *Arch Phys Med Rehabil* 1980;61:351-355.

2. Wolf SL, LeCraw DE, Barton LA: Comparison of motor copy and targeted biofeedback training techniques for restitution of upper extremity function among patients with neurologic disorders. *Phys Therapy* 1989;69:719-735.

3. Wolf SL, Binder-Macleod SA: Electromyographic biofeedback in the physical therapy clinic, in Basmajian JV (ed): *Biofeedback: Principles and Practice for Clinicians*, ed 3. Baltimore, MD, Williams & Wilkins, 1989, pp 91-104.

4. Wolf SL, Binder-Macleod SA: Use of the Krusen Limb Load Monitor to quantify temporal and loading measurements of gait. *Phys Therapy* 1982;62:976-984.

5. Carey PB, Wolf SL, Binder-Macleod SA, et al: Assessing the reliability of measurements from the Krusen Limb Load Monitor to analyze temporal and loading characteristics of normal gait. *Phys Therapy* 1984;64:199-203.

6. Gapsis JJ, Grabois M, Borrell RM, et al: Limb load monitor: Evaluation of a sensory feedback device for controlled weight bearing. *Arch Phys Med Rehabil* 1982;63:38-41.

7. Wannstedt G, Craik RL: Clinical evaluation of a sensory feedback device: The limb load monitor. *Bull Prosthet Res* 1978;Spring:8-49.

8. Wannstedt GT, Herman RM: Use of augmented sensory feedback to achieve symmetrical standing. *Phys Therapy* 1978;58:553-559.

9. Fernie G, Holden J, Soto M: Biofeedback training of knee control in the above-knee amputee. *Am J Phys Med* 1978;57:161-166.

10. Gauthier-Gagnon C, St. Pierre D, Drouin G, et al: Augmented sensory feedback in the early training of standing balance of below-knee amputees. *Physiotherapy (Can)* 1986;38:137-142.

11. *Simplified Taijiquan*, rev ed. Compiled by China Sports Editorial Board. Beijing, China, China Publications Center, 1983, vol. 1.

Chapter 13

A Passive Protective Device to Prevent Hip Fracture From Falls in the Elderly

Jeffrey C. Huston, PhD
Michael S. Sellberg, MS
Carolyn Kundel, PhD
Elizabeth Callan, MS

Introduction

Falling: The Problem

Unintentional falls are the leading cause of injury and loss of independence among the elderly in the United States. Each year, 25% of all persons 65 to 74 years of age and 30% or more of those age 75 or older report a fall.[1] In nursing homes, annual rates are reportedly between 0.6 to 3.6 falls per bed.[2] Ten percent to 20% of falls result in serious injury, and 2% to 6% result in fractures.[3] Although 11,733 deaths were attributed to falls and fall-related injuries in 1987, the actual number of deaths in which a fall was a contributing factor may be much higher.[4] While most falls do not result in serious physical injuries or death, they are often associated with loss of confidence in ability to function independently; restriction of physical and social activities; speech, language, and cognitive disorders; increased dependence; and increased need for long-term care.

In 1985, the total lifetime costs attributed to falls was an estimated $37.3 billion.[1] The lifetime cost of injury for people age 65 and older is estimated to be $14.9 billion, of which nearly $10 billion can be attributed to falls.[1] With growing recognition of the costs of falls and related injuries, the Public Health Service (PHS) of the U.S. Department of Health and Human Services (DHHS) has recently targeted the reduction of falls among older Americans as a major public health objective in its national strategy for significantly improving the health of the nation as discussed in the book, *Healthy People 2000: National Health Promotion and Disease Prevention Objectives*. The specific goal is to "reduce deaths from falls and fall-related injuries to no more than 2.3 per 100,000 people, age-adjusted baseline: 2.7 per 100,000."[4]

Hip Fractures: The Result

An estimated 200,000 hip fractures occur in the elderly each year in the United States.[5] In many patients, fracture of the femur is just the beginning. Sometimes complications develop that may result in death. Only 25% of the elderly who sustain proximal femur fractures fully recover; 20% die.[6] For those who do survive, entrance into a care facility or caregiver assistance is often required. Possibly the most tragic consequence from an injury resulting from a fall is loss of independence and activity, which may lead to a more rapid deterioration of general health.

As of 1982, the elderly comprised only 11% of the United States population while sustaining 70% of all fatalities resulting from falling.[7] As the elderly population percentage continues to increase, fatalities resulting from falls are reaching epidemic levels. The National Hospital Discharge Survey indicates that age-adjusted incidence rates for hip fractures have actually been increasing recently for men and women.[8] Because of the increase in hip fracture rates and the threat to the nation's health, the PHS also specifically targets hip fractures in *Healthy People 2000*: "Reduce hip fractures among people aged 65 and older so that hospitalizations for this condition are no more than 607 per 100,000, baseline: 714 per 100,000 in 1988."[4]

Justification for a Passive Protective Device

Because the factors involved with aging and increased susceptibility to falls are not fully understood, it is now imperative to develop interventions designed to prevent injuries from falls. In the past, hip fracture research has focused on the assessment of in vivo fracture risk[9-11] and the certain therapeutic regimens designed to lessen the impact of factors associated with this risk, such as retarding bone loss.[12] While identifying risk factors, developing successful methods for retarding bone loss, and designing regimens to prevent falls will no doubt be clinically beneficial, the alarming severity of the hip fracture epidemic mandates an immediate passive protective device to shield the hip from the high-impact forces occurring during an accidental fall.

The design objectives for the hip pad protective device focused on two key aspects involved with proximal femur fracture resulting from an accidental fall: (1) the redistribution of dangerous point impact loads away from the greater trochanter into the surrounding soft tissues; and (2) the absorption of a significant amount of the energy generated during a fall. This protection must be provided passively, meaning that once a person dons the hip pad garment, it is not necessary to take any action to receive the protection. The design approach for this device can be justified in recent literature. Hayes and associates[13] report that most hip fractures result when patients fall to the side, land directly on the hip, and do not use their outstretched hand to break the fall. It has also been suggested that energy absorbed during falling and impact, rather than bone strength, appears to be a dominant factor in the biomechanics of hip fracture.[14] Finally, a recent study by Robinovitch and associates[15] concludes that increased soft-tissue thickness over the greater trochanter reduces the "effective stiffness" of the body's soft tissue and subsequently reduces peak impact force to the femur.

Hip Pad Protective Device Development

Development of a device to protect the elderly from hip cractures resulting from falls began at Iowa State University in 1987. A first-generation prototype hip pad protective garment has been developed and used in various clinical trials. The hip pad (approximately 6 in long and 4 in wide) consists of two 3/8-in thick pieces of closed hell polyethylene foam (Minicel T-300) enclosing a 1/10-in high-density polyethylene molded plastic insert. The hip pads are then inserted into side pockets of the garment that hold them in the proper position.

The greater trochanter is a substantial bony prominence and will generally strike the floor or object directly or indirectly in a sideways fall. When the greater trochanter strikes an object, the point impact load causes high bending stresses in the proximal femur because the femur is constrained from moving by the pelvis. These high bending stresses are ultimately the cause of the fracture. By using stress risers, the plastic insert redirects the point impact load away from the greater trochanter and into the surrounding soft tissues. By reducing the point impact load, the bending stresses are lowered, and the risk of fracture is therefore reduced.

To reduce the impact energy of the fall, closed cell polyethylene foam is combined with the plastic insert. In a feasibility study, Turner[16] tested a variety of foams and packing materials for energy absorption. Minicel T-300 was chosen for the design because of its combination of energy absorption, manufacturability, durability, and washability.

The hip pad garment was designed to keep the hip pads positioned over the region of the greater trochanter while providing the maximum amount of comfort for use with the elderly. The garment is constructed from a lightweight, stretchy, 90% cotton, 10% spandex knit that minimizes skin irritation and also provides good breathability.

The garment is currently made in three styles: a female pull-on style, a male pull-on with fly front, and a crotchless style for subjects with incontinence. The open crotch garment is secured into place using Velcro leg closures. Using data from the first year of clinical studies, the garment is now being produced in one of seven sizes. Individual measurements are still taken from every subject and minor alterations are sometimes required.

The garment was tested for washability, durability, and stretch-ability using existing test procedures in the Iowa State University Department of Textiles and Clothing. The garment proved to be extremely tough and durable, yet remained comfortable. Because ease of care is also a significant issue with the elderly, it is noteworthy that tests showed the pads need not be removed from the garment for washing. No significant breakdown of fabric or pad material was recorded during durability testing.

Clinical Evaluation

The clinical evaluation of the hip pad protective garment has been part of a national gerontology study investigating ways to reduce frailty and injuries in the elderly. The study, entitled "Frailty and Injuries: Cooperative Studies of Intervention Techniques" (FICSIT)[17] includes eight sites across the country. The hip pad protective garment being evaluated by the Iowa site (the University of Iowa and Iowa State University) is the only intervention focusing on preventing injury from an accidental fall; the other sites are focusing on accident prevention.[18]

Preliminary Wearability Studies

Two initial clinical wearability studies were performed in nursing homes. Half of the subjects were given 1-in thick pads (1/16-in plastic insert), and the other half were given a thinner 1/2-in pad (1/8-in plastic insert). Subjects were surveyed concerning the comfort, fit, appearance, ease of use, etc., of the hip pad garment.

Changes to the original garment were made: elastic was added to the waistline to prevent the garment from slipping, and the Velcro leg closures were moved from the inner thigh to the front to prevent possible irritation. The thinner hip pad was preferred, but further laboratory testing was required before reducing the overall thickness of the pad.

Compliance Studies

Phase I (April 1990 to February 1991) of the clinical studies began with evaluation of the comfort and wearability of the hip pad garment and pilot studies of nursing home residents. Because of insufficient subject numbers and an initially low acceptance rate (34% compliance rate), the original clinical study of the effectiveness of the hip pad garment evolved into a compliance study. The biggest result obtained in the first year was a definite positive correlation between compliance and cognitive status. Subjects who were mentally alert and aware were more likely to wear the protective garment.

Phase II of the study (March 1991 to February 1992) concentrated on improving compliance with more active, cognitive community-dwelling elderly patients. A run-in technique was also implemented in 64 patients, allowing them to wear the garment without the pads for three days. Once the subjects had adjusted to the garments, the pads were inserted on the fourth day. Participants or their caretakers were asked to record hours of actual wear per day. A measure of compliance was calculated based on self-report diary entries and spot-check telephone calls and visits. The overall compliance rate during waking hours was 80%, with a range of 17% to 99%. Compliance was higher for males, persons with previous fall injuries or greater fear of falling, and persons with fewer cognitive impairments. Phase III of the study is currently in progress and has again focused on compliance. However, this study has included patients who are cognitively impaired, patients with Parkinson's disease, and elderly patients who are generally less active. The compliance rate so far in Phase III has averaged a little over 80%.

Garment Surveys

In an attempt to improve compliance, extensive surveys designed to assess the perceived fit, comfort, utility, safety, and appearance of the garment were conducted during Phase II of the clinical studies. The questionnaire included items on a five-point Likert scale and open-ended questions. Forty-one usable questionnaires were returned, resulting in a 64% response rate, which is acceptable considering the occurrence of age-related illness and mortality in this population. The sex distribution of the sample was 68% female and 32% male. The mean age was 74, with a range of 59 to 89 years. Seventy-one percent of the respondents lived in their own homes and 29% lived in retirement centers or care facilities.

Fit　　Perceptions of fit were assessed at the waist, hip, leg, and crotch using the scale shown in Table 1. Frequency distributions showed that the majority of participants rated each fit characteristic favorably, as shown by these percentages.

Participants also rated the extent to which they thought the hip pad garment affected the fit of their regular clothing. As Table 2 shows, respondents' ratings were mixed. A comparison of the frequency distributions by sex suggests that women tended to think the hip pad garment interfered more with their regular clothing than did men.

Comfort　　Comfort was assessed both by garment characteristics and by comfort during specific activities. The garment characteristics of fabric hand, fabric weight, and garment weight all received highly favorable ratings, with no notable differences by sex. As shown in Figure 1, responses were mixed on the characteristic of thermal comfort, with most participants responding that the garment was somewhat warm or too warm. This was a common complaint throughout the trial. Most participants wore the garment over their underwear.

Table 1 Perceptions of fit

Scale	Waist	Hip	Leg	Crotch
Very loose	4.9%	2.4%	14.6%	2.7%
Loose	17.1%	2.4%	56.1%	5.4%
Just right	61.0%	70.7%	24.4%	78.4%
Tight	17.0%	22.0%	4.9%	10.8%
Very tight	0.0%	2.4%	0.0%	2.7%

Table 2 Garment effect on fit of regular clothing

Scale	Frequency	Total (%)	Women (%)	Men (%)
Very much	8	20.0	28.6	0.0
Moderately	17	42.5	39.2	50.0
Uncertain	1	2.5	3.6	0.0
Hardly at all	14	35.0	28.6	50.0
Not at all	0	0.0	0.0	0.0

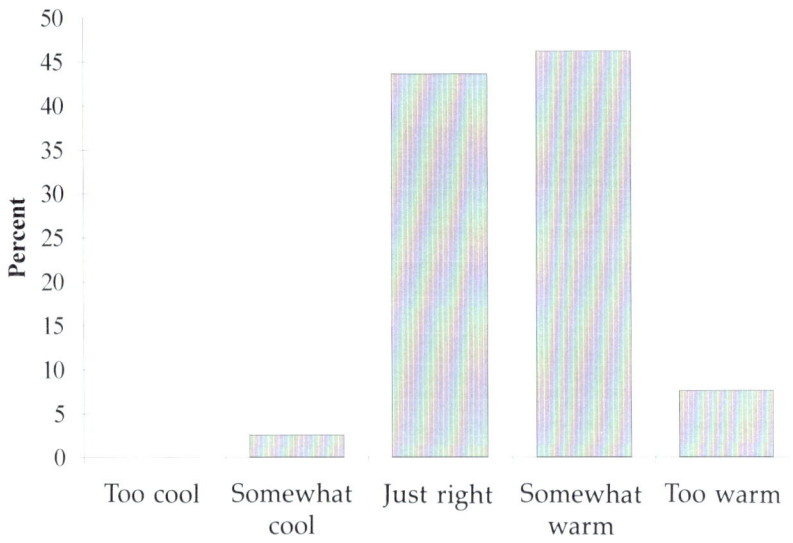

Fig. 1 *Thermal comfort. (Reproduced with permission from Sellberg MS, Huston JC, Kruger DH: The development of a passive protective device for the elderly to prevent hip fractures from accidental falls. Adv Bioeng 1992;22:505-508.)*

Because responses suggested that the garment may be too warm, a lighter weight knit fabric was used in Trial III.

For comfort during specific activities, the majority of the participants gave highly favorable ratings to comfort while sitting and while walking. Seventy percent of the participants chose not to wear the garment to bed, so accurate assessment of comfort while sleeping was not possible. When asked to assess overall comfort, 10% of the respondents rated the garment as excellent, 56% thought it was good, 30% said it was fair, and only 3% rated it as poor.

Utility   Utility of the garment was assessed by three functional use aspects: how easy it was for participants to put the garment on, take the garment off, and use the bathroom with the garment. In addition, how the garment affected participants' level of daily activity was also measured.

As the frequency distribution in Figure 2 shows, these measures received favorable ratings overall. However, 17% of the participants, some of whom had severe arthritis in their hands, thought that putting the garment on was difficult. For these participants, loops made from twill tape were sewn on the inside of their garments to make them easier to grip and to pull on. In terms of toileting, 28% of the respondents thought toileting was difficult. For men, the problem was related to design. Several men complained that the fly-front opening was too high; as a result, the fly opening has been lowered.

Comments from women suggest that their problem with toileting is related to urgency. However, these women are not incontinent and refuse to wear the crotchless style garment that would allow for quicker toileting. One possible solution to this problem is to discourage these women from wearing additional layers of clothing, such as girdles and slips. One subject has stopped wearing her girdle and has requested garters be sewn onto her hip pad garment.

Safety   Safety assessments focused on a subject's fear of falling and the perception of safety while wearing the hip pad. Surprisingly, frail elderly participants tended to be less fearful of falling than expected, as shown in Figure 3. Distributions by sex suggest that women were only slightly more fearful than men. However, chi-square results showed no difference by sex in fear of falling.

Participants were then asked to rate how safe they felt from sustaining a hip fracture under two conditions: when wearing the hip pad garment and without it. As shown in Table 3, most of the respondents were uncertain about their feelings of safety in both instances, and wearing the hip pad garment seemed to increase feelings of safety only slightly.

Appearance   Respondents were asked to make self-evaluations of satisfaction with their physical appearance with and without the hip pad garment in place. As Table 4 shows, the frequency distribution suggests a decrease in satisfaction ratings when wearing the garment. Women expressed more dissatisfaction with appearance than men.

Overall, men tended to give higher self-evaluations on physical appearance than did women. Kappa tests revealed high levels of agreement between satisfaction with physical appearance while

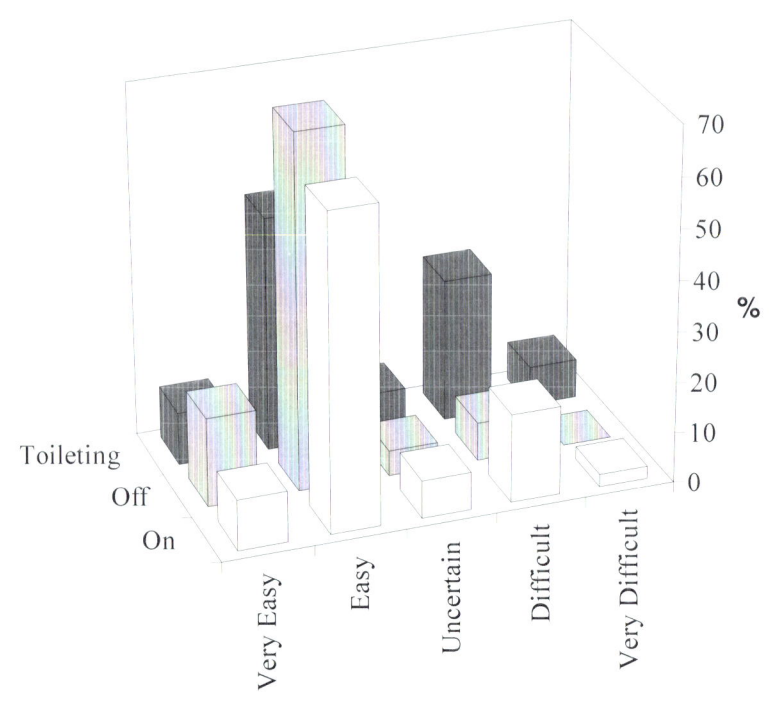

Fig. 2 *Utility functions.*

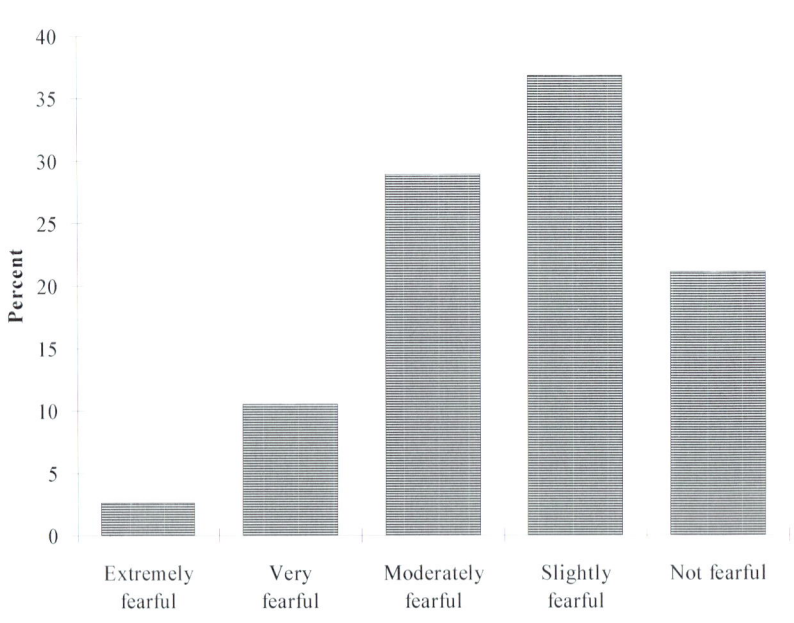

Fig. 3 *Fear of falling.*

Table 3 Safety

Scale	Without the Hip Pads		With the Hip Pads	
	Frequency	Percent	Frequency	Percent
Very safe	4	17.1	3	9.1
Safe	8	22.2	12	36.4
Uncertain	21	58.3	17	51.1
Unsafe	3	8.3	1	3.0
Very unsafe	0	0.0	0	0.0

Table 4 Physical appearance

Scale	Without the Hip Pads		With the Hip Pads	
	Frequency	Percent	Frequency	Percent
Very satisfied	6	15.4	1	2.6
Satisfied	19	48.7	14	35.9
Uncertain	5	12.8	10	25.6
Dissatisfied	9	23.1	12	30.8
Very dissatisfied	0	0.0	2	5.1

wearing the hip pad garment and when not wearing it. In other words, the majority of respondents tended to report the same level of satisfaction with appearance both with and without the hip pad garment.

Falls

Over 36 falls occurred during Phase II. In 27 (75%) of these falls, the subjects were wearing the hip pads. In seven instances, subjects reported falling directly on the hip pad. No hip fractures or serious hip injuries were reported. In two of the subjects, the fall impact was directly onto a previously fractured hip. Both subjects had minor bruising and believed that the hip pad prevented a hip fracture. These two cases are particularly encouraging, considering the weakened condition of bone after fracture. A third subject impacted the hip pad directly onto a piece of shop iron. The hip pad also effectively shielded the greater trochanter from this severe point load situation.

So far in Phase III, 54 falls have occurred. The hip pad was worn in 45 of these falls, an 83% compliance rate. Twelve of the 45 reported falls with hip pads resulted in a direct impact on the greater trochanter (covered by the hip pad). No fractures or serious injuries were reported in any of these falls. Three of these 12 falls were directly on a previously fractured hip, including one case in which a man fell from a stepladder onto his once broken hip. The hip pad garment successfully protected the patients in all these cases. The number of falls for Phases II and III is summarized in Figure 4.

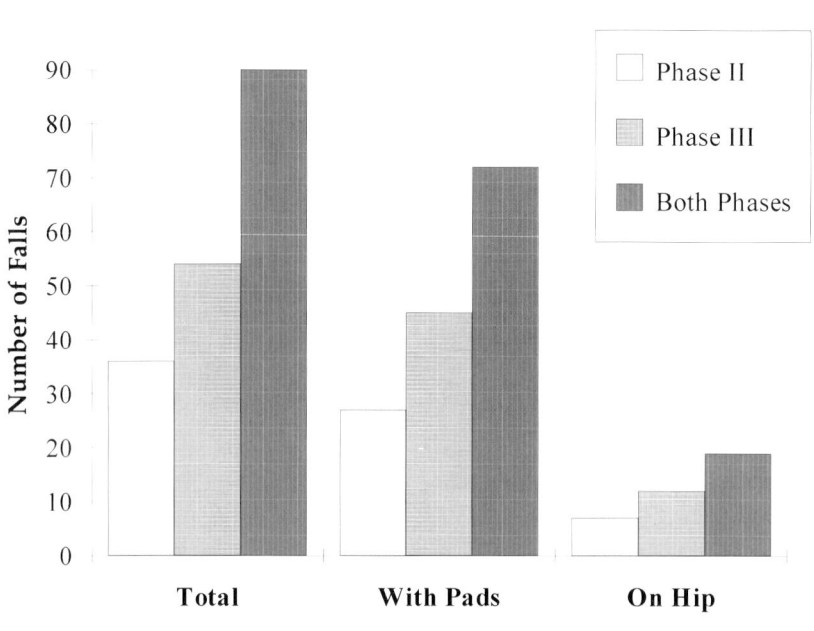

Fig. 4 *Falls, Phases II and III.*

Laboratory Testing of the Hip Pad

Preliminary Low Energy Impact Testing

Low energy impact testing of the 1-in (1/16-in plastic insert) hip pad were conducted. A pendulum testing device equipped with a single impact force transducer (PCB 200A05) was used to measure the percent reduction in peak impact force. With the force transducer embedded in the pendulum (weight = 145 N), which was curved to duplicate soft tissue curvature around the proximal femur, a flat steel plate covered with carpet was struck with and without the pads from varying heights. A Tektronix 2201 digital oscilloscope was used to record and store the force-time history. Each stored signal was then transferred using Tektronix Grabber software to a Zenith 80286 laptop computer via the RS-232 serial port. The average peak impact force of approximately 1,540 N was reduced 40 times to an average of 36 N by the 1-in pad.

Because compliance was low and many subjects complained that the 1-in pads were too thick, thinner pads were developed. To support the use of these thinner pads, additional low energy impact testing was conducted. The 1/2-in thick pad with 1/8-in plastic insert and a 3/4-in thick pad with 1/8-in plastic insert were tested. The 1/2-in pad reduced an average peak load of 1,538 N (345.8 lb) over 30 times to an average of 46 N, while the 3/4-in pad reduced the same peak

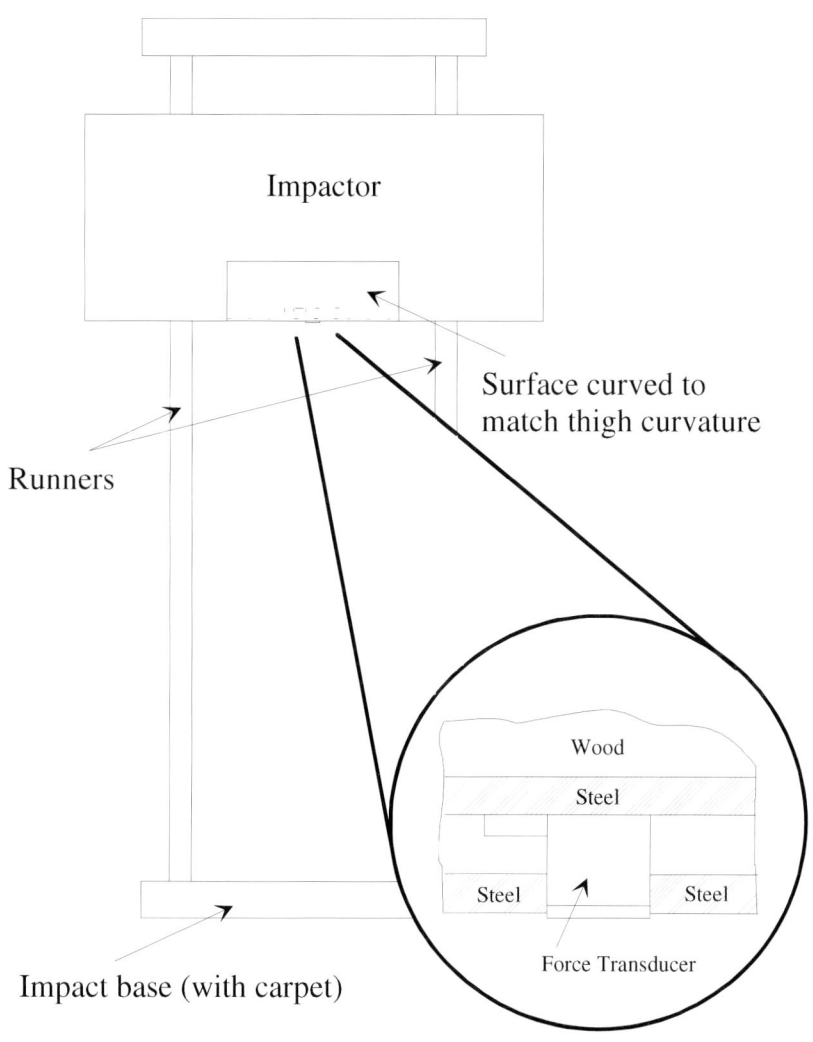

Impactor

Surface curved to match thigh curvature

Runners

Wood

Steel

Steel

Steel

Force Transducer

Impact base (with carpet)

Fig. 5 *High energy impact tester.*

load 35 times to an average of 43 N (9.7 lb). With these test results and the results from the wearability survey, the decision was made to use the 3/4-in thick pad, but substitute a 1/10-in plastic insert for the 1/8-in plastic insert for future clinical studies.

High Energy Impact Testing

To duplicate the potential energy in a typical fall and to provide higher impact forces, a testing device was constructed as shown in Figure 5. The impact force transducer and data acquisition system from the pendulum tester are used with this new device. Weights were added to the impactor head until the total drop weight equaled 357 N (80.2 lb). This weight was chosen to approximately match the effective moving masses reported by Robinovitch and associates[15] in their pelvis release experiments. The impactor was designed with an embedded force transducer and curvature duplicating the soft tissue surrounding the proximal femur.

The impactor was dropped from three drop heights (0.30 m = 1 ft, 0.61 m = 2 ft, and 0.91m = 3 ft creating energy levels of 108.8 J, 217.6 J, and 326.4 J, respectively) with and without the hip pads onto the steel impact base, which was covered with a 3/4-in piece of ply-

Table 5 Baseline and hip pad impact forces

| | Impact Forces (N)* | | | | | | | |
| | Baseline | | | | 3/4-Inch Hip Pad | | | |
Energy Level (J)	Avg	SD	Min	Max	Avg	SD	Min	Max
108.8	2085.10	143.52	2313.08	1868.25	309.71	134.29	604.96	151.24
217.6	3553.02	147.41	3736.51	3291.68	2124.03	343.53	2668.93	1690.32
326.4	4620.59	99.29	4804.08	4492.70	2919.15	342.86	3558.58	2579.97

*Avg, average; SD, standard deviation; min, minimum; max, maximum.

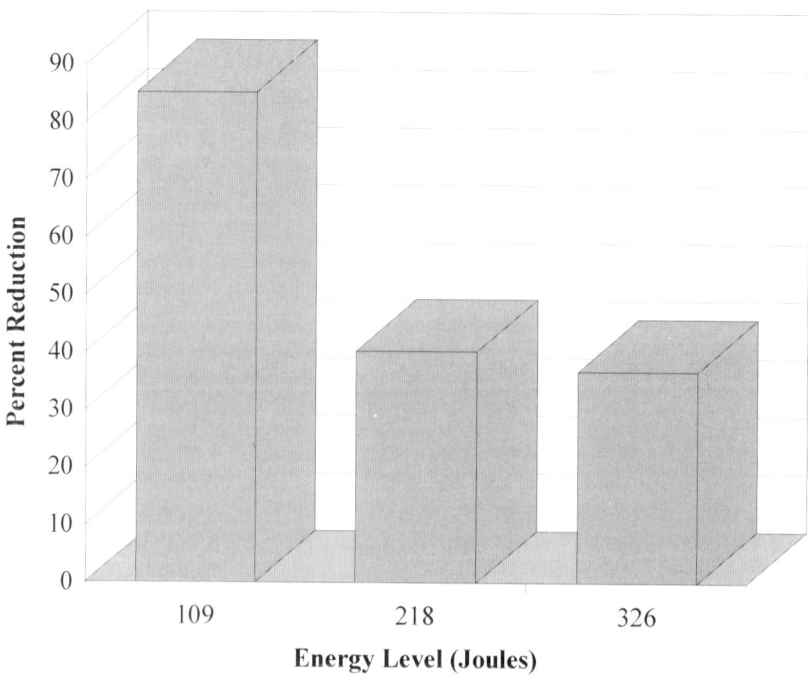

Fig. 6 *Average percent reduction in peak impact force.*

wood and 1/4-in of carpet. The maximum theoretic velocities from each of the heights were 2.45 m/s from 0.30 m, 3.26 m/s from 0.61 m, and 4.24 m/s from the 0.91 m. Eight sets of runs without the pad (baseline) and with the 3/4-in pads were conducted from each height. The average, maximum, and minimum impact forces and the standard deviation for both the baseline and the hip pads are presented in Table 5.

Figure 6, which shows the average percent reduction in impact force, represents the percentage of the impact load that is absorbed and distributed away from the embedded force transducer by the hip pad. At the highest energy level (326.4 J), the hip pad reduces the baseline impact force 36.82%. More reduction was achieved at the smaller energy levels, 40.22% at 217.6 J and 85.15% at 326.4 J.

Summary

While the test apparatus does not accurately represent the complex human kinematics nor in vivo biomechanics of a fall, it does provide a severe laboratory test for the hip pads. While the velocity of impact of a real fall may be slowed by neurologic reactions, by "breaking the fall" with limbs, or by striking other objects before the proximal femur impacts the floor, the impact tester provides a free fall drop of a concentrated mass. This free falling mass has no surrounding soft tissue and is embedded with a small diameter (compared to the greater trochanter) force transducer; therefore, it provides more severe point loading characteristics than the actual in vivo load history from a fall.

Laboratory tests show that the hip pads significantly reduce the baseline impact force. Lotz and Hayes[14] have shown fracture loads for the proximal femur of cadavers to be in the range of 778 N to 4093 N. The average baseline impact forces at all three heights were well within this range, with the average force of 4620 N at 0.91-m drop height exceeding this range. Weber and associates[19] have shown that loading rates are important in determining fracture force. With a slow loading rate of 0.7 mm/s, their fracture load was 2933 N. A medium loading rate of 14 mm/s yielded a fracture force of 3505 N and the fastest load rate of 4 m/s gave the highest fracture force of 6017 N. While the maximum average impact load of 4620 N is lower than Weber and associates' maximum, the tester still offers a severe test because of the theoretical velocity of 4.24 m/s at the 0.91-m drop height.

As Table 5 shows, considerable variability in the impact forces with the hip pads exists, mainly because of the manufacturing process currently used for the prototypes. The plastic inserts and the top foam piece are compression molded by hand, yielding a slightly different pad each time. After further laboratory and clinical testing of the hip pad device, a full-scale injection molding process will be developed that will eliminate this current quality control problem. While no overall conclusions can be drawn at this time concerning the hip pads' effectiveness in reducing the impact below the fracture threshold, it does appear that from a height of 0.30 m the hip pads eliminate the hip fracture risk.

Future work includes extending the scope of both laboratory and clinical testing of the device. A nationwide clinical study is being planned to generate the numbers (3,000 to 5,000 subjects) needed to prove with statistical significance the hip pad's clinical effectiveness. Alternate hip pad designs are being evaluated, including different plastics and new foams. Extensive work is being planned in the areas of fall dynamics and simulation. Studies in this area can shed light onto possible impact force histories that can be used in conjunction with finite element models of the hip pad, pelvis, and femur to optimize the hip pad design.

Acknowledgments

Initial design and prototype work has been funded by Iowa State University, Ames, Iowa, and Mercy Medical Center, Des Moines, Iowa. Clinical studies and minor device modifications have been supported by NIH grant NR02638-03 through the University of Iowa Department of Preventive Medicine, Dr. Robert Wallace, Principal Investigator, and Jo Ross, Project Director.

References

1. National Injury Control Conference: Position Papers from the Third National Injury Control Conference: *Setting the National Agenda for Injury Control in the 1990s.* Atlanta, GA, Department of Health and Human Services, 1992.

2. Perry BC: Falls among the elderly: A review of the methods and conclusions of epidemiologic studies. *J Am Geriatr Soc* 1982;30:367-371.

3. Rubenstein LZ, Robbins AS, Schulman BL, et al: Falls and instability in the elderly. *J Am Geriatr Soc* 1988;36:266-278.

4. U.S. Public Health Service: *Healthy People 2000: National Health Promotion and Disease Prevention Objectives.* Washington, DC, U.S. Department of Health and Human Services, 1990, DHHS Pub. No. (PHS) 91-50212.

5. National Center for Health Statistics: *Health Statistics on Older Persons, United States, 1986.* U.S. Department of Health and Human Services, Hyattsville, MD, 1987, DHHS Publication No. (PHS) 87-1409.

6. Hofeldt F: Proximal femoral fractures. *Clin Orthop* 1987;218:12-18.

7. Metropolitan Life Insurance Company: Mortality from leading types of accidents (statistical bulletin). New York, NY, Metropolitan Life Insurance Company, 1982.

8. Rodriguez JG, Sattin RW, Waxweiler RJ: Incidence of hip fractures, United States, 1970-1983. *Am J Prev Med* 1989;5:175-181.

9. Mizrahi J, Margulies JY, Leichter I, et al: Fracture of the human femoral neck: Effect of density of the cancellous core. *J Biomed Eng* 1984;6:56-62.

10. Phillips JR, Williams JF, Melick RA: Prediction of the strength of the neck of femur from its radiological appearance. *Biomed Eng* 1975;10:367-372.

11. Vose GP, Mack PB: Roentgenologic assessment of femoral neck density as related to fracturing. *Am J Roentgenol* 1963;89:1296-1301.

12. Paganini-Hill A, Ross RK, Gerkins VR, et al: Menopausal estrogen therapy and hip fracture. *Ann Intern Med* 1981;95:28-31.

13. Hayes WC, Myers ER, Morris JN, et al: Fall biomechanics as determinants of osteoporotic hip fracture risk, in Deluca HF, Mazess R (eds): *Osteoporosis: Physiologic Basis, Assessment, and Treatment: Proceedings of the 19th Steenbock Symposium*, held June 5, 1989 at the University of Wisconsin. New York, NY, Elsevier Science Publishing Co, 1990, p 40.

14. Lotz JC, Hayes WC: The use of quantitative computed tomography to estimate risk of fracture of the hip from falls. *J Bone Joint Surg* 1990;72A:689-700.

15. Robinovitch SN, Hayes WC, McMahon TA: Prediction of femoral impact forces in falls on the hip. *J Biomech Eng* 1991;113:366-374.

16. Turner J: *Use of Protective Hip Pads to Prevent or Reduce Hip Injury: A Feasibility Study*. Ames, IA, Iowa State University, 1988. Thesis.

17. Wallace RB, Ross JE, Huston JC, et al: Iowa FICSIT trial: The feasibility of elderly wearing a hip joint protective garment to reduce hip fractures. *J Am Geriatr Soc* 1993;41:338-340.

18. Ross JC, Maas ML, Huston JC, et al: Evaluation of two interventions to reduce falls and fall injuries: The challenge of hip pads and individualized elimination rounds, in Funk SG, Tornquist EM, Champagne MT, et al (eds): *Key Aspects of Elder Care: Managing Falls, Incontinence, and Cognitive Impairment*. New York, NY, Springer Publishing Co, 1992, chap 10, pp 97-103.

19. Weber TG, Yang KH, Woo R, et al: Proximal femur strength: Correlation of the rate of loading and bone mineral density. *Adv Bioeng* 1992;BED-Vol 22:111-114.

Overview and Future Directions for Research

David F. Apple, Jr., MD
Wilson C. Hayes, PhD

Etiology

Twelve million falls occur annually, compared with 4 million motor vehicle accidents. These falls cause over 280,000 fractured hips, resulting in health care costs of over $10 billion. Intrinsic factors associated with falls causing fractured hips are age and sex, with women older than 70 years most at risk. Additional intrinsic factors include balance and vision problems, lower extremity muscle weakness, and side effects from medications. Except for age and sex, interventions are available to many of these factors. Extrinsic factors associated with falls, such as stairs, lighting, rugs, crutches, and canes, are related to the patient's environment.

The interrelations between intrinsic and extrinsic factors need clarification. More study is needed so that the most efficacious and cost-effective intervention is developed. One of the most pressing needs is effective and practical evaluation tools to screen those patients most at risk for falls and for hip fractures when a fall occurs.

Treatment

The goal of the orthopaedic surgeon should be to restore the patient to a prefracture level of function. All hip fractures require treatment, and most require surgery. The patient who is best served by nonsurgical treatment needs to be identified. In addition, fracture treatment is a small part of the total management of the patient, and this management should be undertaken with a team approach, including not only the orthopaedic surgeon but a gerontologist, primary care physician, social worker, physical therapist, and perhaps others.

Multicenter studies should be performed to further clarify the philosophy of treatment and implant selection (for example, pinning versus use of a primary prosthesis in treating a subcapital fracture and the complications that sometimes result with both methods). This would identify which fracture to fix and when. Development of a clinical pathway for treatment of hip fractures would also be helpful. The effect that health care policy, especially as it relates to financing, will have on the total treatment of the elderly patient with a hip fracture is cause for concern.

Prevention

Prevention strategies are in their early stages of development, and more study is needed to decrease the risk of fractures in high-risk patients. Areas currently under investigation are trochanteric padding, conventional aerobic and resistance exercise programs, alternative exercise endeavors such as Tai Chi and balance training, along with more conventional approaches to the treatment of osteoporosis. Further study of the most commonly used drugs in geriatrics and their role in creating falls could lead to identifying low-risk alternative drugs. More community-based programs need to be developed to study the effectiveness of these intervention efforts outside of nursing homes.

Future Directions

1. Reimbursement patterns should be influenced so that the care of an elderly patient with a fractured hip is extended beyond just fracture management.
2. Government agencies such as National Institute of Arthritis and Musculoskeletal and Skin Diseases and Centers for Disease Control and Prevention should be encouraged to fund research on risk studies, treatment outcomes, and prevention strategies.
3. Research partnerships with business and the insurance industry should be developed to analyze both fracture treatment and prevention.
4. Coalitions should be developed with the appropriate organizations, such as the National Institute of Aging, National Institutes of Health, American Association of Retired Persons, National Osteoporosis Foundation, and National Geriatric Society, to help with research and public education, and to help influence health care policy.
5. Public and medical educational programs focusing on the problem of falls and hip fractures in the elderly should be expanded.

Index

Activities of daily living (ADL), 85, 86, 88
Activity level, correlation of, with falls, 48
Age
  as factor in hip fractures, 41, 48
  as factor in injurious falls, 74, 76–77
Agent factors, as risk factor in injurious falls, 79
Alcohol
  as factor in bone loss, 35
  as factor in injurious falls, 79
Arms, failure to extend, as factor in hip fractures, 50, 52
Arthritis, as factor in falls, 108
Austin-Moore hemiarthroplasties, 89
Autogenous bone graft, 100

Balance, as risk factor in falls, 77–78, 108, 110
Balance System (Chattecx Company), 120
Balance training, 144
  assessment of, 124–125
  computerized, 119
  differences between Tai Chi Quan and, 121–122
Basilar neck fractures, 95
Bicycle helmets, use of, 4
Biomechanics of falls and hip fracture in elderly, 41–63
Bipolar hemiarthroplasty, 89
Blacks, intentional injuries among, 2
Blindness, as risk factor for falls, 108
Bone density
  basis of, in defining osteoporosis, 22
  as potential predictor of hip fractures, 22–23
Bone mass, measurement of, as index of risk for hip fractures, 34
Bone weakness, and risk of injury from falls, 10

Calcium, in determining peak bone mass, 35

Cancer, association with hip fracture, 12, 15
Cardiac insufficiency, and dizziness, 20
Centers for Disease Control and Prevention (CDC), role of, in injury prevention, 1–6
Cephalomedullary nails, 102
Chlordiazepoxide, association with falls, 20
Chronic illness
  as risk factor for hip fracture, 9–16
    case-control study, 10–12
  as risk factor in injurious falls, 75, 77
Cochran-Mantel-Haenszel (CMH) statistics, use of, in determination of hip fracture risk, 50–51
Cognitive impairment, association with hip fractures, 12
Compression hip screw, 98
Computerized balance training, 119
Condylocephalic implants, 99

Dementia, as risk factor for falls, 15, 108
Diazepam, association with falls, 20
Disease, as factor in bone loss, 35
Dizziness, as factor in hip fractures, 52

Ender nail, 99
Energies associated with falls, 53–54
Energy content of fall, as factor in hip fractures, 51–52
Environment
  hazards in, as factor in falls, 79, 110
  influence of, on peak bone mass, 35–36
Estrogen
  as factor in bone loss associated with menopause, 35
  as factor in microfracture healing, 28
  in prevention of hip fractures, 29–30
Exercise, as factor in peak bone mass, 35